The Microbiome: Interactions with Organ Systems, Diet, and Genetics

Editor

ROCHELLYS DIAZ HEIJTZ

GASTROENTEROLOGY CLINICS OF NORTH AMERICA

www.gastro.theclinics.com

Consulting Editor
ALAN L. BUCHMAN

September 2019 • Volume 48 • Number 3

ELSEVIER

1600 John F. Kennedy Boulevard • Suite 1800 • Philadelphia, Pennsylvania, 19103-2899
http://www.theclinics.com

GASTROENTEROLOGY CLINICS OF NORTH AMERICA Volume 48, Number 3
September 2019 ISSN 0889-8553, ISBN-13: 978-0-323-67900-8

Editor: Kerry Holland
Developmental Editor: Laura Kavanaugh

Gastroenterology Clinics of North America (ISSN 0889-8553) is published quarterly by Elsevier Inc., 360 Park Avenue South, New York, NY 10010-1710. Months of issue are March, June, September, and December. Business and Editorial Offices: 1600 John F. Kennedy Blvd., Suite 1800, Philadelphia, PA 19103-2899. Customer Service Office: 6277 Sea Harbor Drive, Orlando, FL 32887-4800. Periodicals postage paid at New York, NY and additional mailing offices. Subscription prices are $361.00 per year (US individuals), $100.00 per year (US students), $692.00 per year (US institutions), $387.00 per year (Canadian individuals), $220.00 per year (Canadian students), $849.00 per year (Canadian institutions), $463.00 per year (international individuals), $220.00 per year (international students), and $849.00 per year (international institutions). Foreign air speed delivery is included in all *Clinics* subscription prices. All prices are subject to change without notice. **POSTMASTER**: Send address changes to *Gastroenterology Clinics of North America*, Elsevier Health Sciences Division, Subscription Customer Service, 3251 Riverport Lane, Maryland Heights, MO 63043. **Telephone: 1-800-654-2452 (U.S. and Canada); 314-447-8871 (outside U.S. and Canada). Fax: 314-447-8029. E-mail: journalscustomerservice-usa@elsevier.com (for print support); journalsonlinesupport-usa@elsevier.com (for online support).**

Reprints. For copies of 100 or more, of articles in this publication, please contact the Commercial Reprints Department, Elsevier Inc., 360 Part Avenue South, New York, New York 10010-1710. Tel. 212-633-3874, Fax: 212-633-3820, E-mail: reprints@elsevier.com.

Gastroenterology Clinics of North America is also published in Italian by Il Pensiero Scientifico Editore, Rome, Italy; and in Portuguese by Interlivros Edicoes Ltda., Rua Commandante Coelho 1085, 21250 Cordovil, Rio de Janeiro, Brazil.

Gastroenterology Clinics of North America is covered in *MEDLINE/PubMed (Index Medicus), Excerpta Medica, Current Contents/Clinical Medicine, Science Citation Index, ISI/BIOMED,* and *BIOSIS*.

Contributors

CONSULTING EDITOR

ALAN L. BUCHMAN, MD, MSPH, FACP, FACN, FACG, AGAF
Medical Director, Health Care Services Corporation, Professor of Clinical Surgery and Medical Director, Intestinal Rehabilitation and Transplant Center, The University of Illinois at Chicago, Chicago, Illinois, USA

EDITOR

ROCHELLYS DIAZ HEIJTZ, PhD
Associate Professor, Department of Neuroscience, Karolinska Institutet, Stockholm, Sweden; Full Professor, INSERM U1239, University of Rouen Normandy, Mont-Saint-Aignan, France

AUTHORS

KJERSTI M. AAGAARD, MD, PhD, FACOG
Henry and Emma Meyer Chair in Obstetrics & Gynecology, Professor & Vice Chair of Research, Obstetrics & Gynecology, Division of Maternal-Fetal Medicine, Medical Scientist Training Program, Translational Biology & Molecular Medicine, Center for Microbiome and Metagenomics Research, Molecular & Human Genetics, Molecular & Cell Biology, Baylor College of Medicine, Houston, Texas, USA

MARIA AMATO, MSc
Department of Human Genetics, Donders Institute for Brain, Cognition and Behaviour, Radboud University Medical Center, Nijmegen, The Netherlands

ALEJANDRO ARIAS-VASQUEZ, PhD
Departments of Human Genetics and Psychiatry, Donders Institute for Brain, Cognition and Behaviour, Radboud University Medical Center, Nijmegen, The Netherlands

BEATRIZ PEÑALVER BERNABÉ, PhD
Aronld O. Beckman Postdoctoral Fellow, Microbiome Center, University of Chicago, Chicago, Illinois, USA

MIRJAM BLOEMENDAAL, PhD
Department of Psychiatry, Donders Institute for Brain, Cognition and Behaviour, Radboud University Medical Center, Nijmegen, The Netherlands

NELE BRUSSELAERS, MD, MSc, PhD
Associate Professor, Centre for Translational Microbiome Research, Department of Microbiology, Tumor and Cell Biology, Karolinska Institutet, Science for Life Laboratory, Stockholm, Sweden

CYNTHIA M. BULIK, PhD
University of North Carolina at Chapel Hill, Chapel Hill, North Carolina, USA

Recently it has become clear that the microbial communities in our respiratory system and our gut, as well as on our skin, may play a key role in shaping our physiology, and influencing our health. We are only beginning to understand the mechanisms by which the human microbiota may be regulating the immune system, and sudden changes in the composition of the microbiota may have profound effects, linked with an increased risk of developing chronic inflammatory disorders, including allergies.

The gut microbiota, acting via the gut-brain axis, modulates key neurobiological systems that are dysregulated in stress-related disorders. Preclinical studies show that the gut microbiota exerts an influence over neuroimmune and neuroendocrine signaling pathways, in addition to epigenetic modification, neurogenesis, and neurotransmission. In humans, preliminary evidence suggests that the gut microbiota profile is altered in depression. The full impact of microbiota-based treatments, at different neurodevelopmental time points, has yet to be fully explored. The integration of the gut microbiota, as a mediator, in the complex trajectory of depression, may enhance the possibility of personalized precision psychiatry.

Genetic and environmental factors play a role in the cause and development of attention–deficit/hyperactivity disorder (ADHD). Recent studies have suggested an important role of the gut-brain axis (GBA) and intestinal microbiota in modulating the risk of ADHD. Here, the authors provide a brief overview of the clinical and biological picture of ADHD and how the GBA could be involved in its cause. They discuss key biological mechanisms involved in the GBA and how these may increase the risk of developing ADHD. Understanding these mechanisms may help to characterize novel treatment options via identification of disease biomarkers.

Perinatal mood and anxiety disorders (PMAD) have significant negative impacts on mother and child, yet treatments are limited. Adequate nutrition during the perinatal period is essential to maternal and infant health, including maternal mental health and the child's neurologic and neuropsychiatric development. Nutrition holds promise to improve prevention and treatment of PMAD. The ability to manipulate the gut microbiota composition and structure through host nutrition and to harness the gut microbes for improved individualized nutrition may be an important new direction for prevention and treatment of PMAD, thus improving the mental health of mother and child.

The Microbiota and Pancreatic Cancer

Tomasz M. Karpiński

Pancreatic cancer is one of the most lethal diseases. In pancreatic cancer development and progression, genetic (gene mutations and activation of oncogenes) and environmental factors (smoking, alcohol consumption, type 2 diabetes mellitus, obesity) play an essential role. Recently, molecular studies revealed that dysbiosis of microbiota also has influence on cancer development. Research indicates that bacteria and viruses can lead to chronic inflammation, antiapoptotic changes, cell survival, and cell invasion. This review presents bacteria and viruses oncogenic for the pancreas. Possible mechanisms of carcinogenic action are also described.

The Microbiome: Interactions with Organ Systems, Diet, and Genetics

GASTROENTEROLOGY
CLINICS OF NORTH AMERICA

SERIES OF RELATED INTEREST

Gastrointestinal Endoscopy Clinics of North America
(Available at: https://www.giendo.theclinics.com)
Clinics in Liver Disease
(Available at: https://www.liver.theclinics.com)

THE CLINICS ARE AVAILABLE ONLINE!
Access your subscription at:
www.theclinics.com

Preface

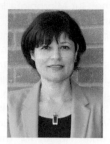

Rochellys Diaz Heijtz, PhD
Editor

Over the last 2 decades, microbiome research has profoundly shaped our perception of human biology and the origin of human diseases. It is now recognized that the microbiome is a critical component of human physiology, and that its disruption or imbalance could contribute to the development and manifestation of common human diseases, including metabolic diseases, inflammatory bowel disease, neurologic and psychiatric conditions, and cancer, among others. The human microbiome, the trillions of indigenous microorganisms (bacteria, bacteriophages, fungi, protozoa, and viruses) that colonize the body and, more specifically, their microbial genomes, is a part of the "human genetic landscape." Studies have demonstrated that these microbes interact with their host and play an essential role in many host physiologic processes, including dietary energy extraction, the production of vitamins, and protection against pathogens. Beyond these traditional functions, microbial colonization has been shown to contribute to the developmental programming of epithelial barrier function, gut homeostasis, and angiogenesis, as well as the development and function of the gut immune system. More recent findings have revealed that the gut microbiome has effects on host physiology and development outside the gastrointestinal system, including the early-life programming of brain circuits involved in the control of emotions, motor activity, and cognitive functions. In recent years, we have begun to unravel the function of microbiomes associated with specific habitats in the human body, and the signaling pathways mediating the complex and dynamic interactions between the microbiome and its host tissues. Our understanding of the role of the microbiome in health and disease is rapidly expanding due to recent technological advances in "Omics" sciences: sequencing, proteomics, and metabolomics, as well as analytical and computational tools for systems biology and integrative analysis. Mounting evidence suggests that the human microbiome can be influenced by many factors, including genetics, diet, age, toxic agents, and drugs.

Microbiome research is inherently and extensively interdisciplinary and thus has integrated skills and knowledge across many disciplines, including immunology, bioinformatics, mathematics, biochemistry, epidemiology, neuroscience, and psychiatry.

Gastroenterol Clin N Am 48 (2019) xi–xii
https://doi.org/10.1016/j.gtc.2019.07.001
0889-8553/19/© 2019 Published by Elsevier Inc.

This special issue on "The Microbiome: Interactions with Organ Systems, Diet, and Genetics" captures some of the progress that has been made in the following areas: 1. Prescribed Drugs and the Microbiome (Nele Brusselaers, Karolinska Institutet, Sweden); 2. Gut-Brain Interactions: Implications for a Role of the Gut Microbiota in the Treatment and Prognosis of Anorexia Nervosa and Comparison to Type I Diabetes (Cynthia M. Bulik, University of North Carolina at Chapel Hill, USA); 3. The Development of the Human Microbiome: Why Moms Matters (Kjersti Agaard, Baylor College of Medicine, USA); 4. The Human Microbiota and its Relationship with Allergies (Nanna Fyhrquist, Karolinska Institutet, Sweden and University of Helsinki, Finland); 5. Mood and Microbes: Gut-to-Brain Communication in Depression (Timothy G. Dinan, University of Cork, Ireland); 6. The Role of the Gut-Brain Axis in Attention-Deficit/Hyperactivity Disorder (Alejandro Arias-Vasquez, Radboud University Medical Centre, The Netherlands); 7. Improving Mental Health for the Mother-Infant Dyad by Nutrition and the Maternal Gut Microbiome (Mary C. Kimmel, University of North Carolina at Chapel Hill, USA); 8. The Microbiota and Pancreatic Cancer (Tomasz M. Karpiński, Poznanń University of Medical Sciences, Poland).

I would like to thank all the authors and all the reviewers who kindly helped and contributed to this special issue.

I hope that this special issue provides new insights into the human microbiome and its interactions with host organ systems and that it stimulates new discussions and research directions in this exciting research field.

Rochellys Diaz Heijtz, PhD
Department of Neuroscience
Karolinska Instituet
171 77 Stockholm, Sweden

INSERM U1239
University of Rouen Normandy
76130 Mont-Saint-Aignan, France

E-mail address:
Rochellys.Heijtz@ki.se

Prescribed Drugs and the Microbiome

Nele Brusselaers, MD, MSc, PhD[a,b,*]

KEYWORDS

- Prescribed drug use • Microbiome • Medication • Prescribing • Translational
- Pharmacomicrobiomics

KEY POINTS

- Prescribed drug use is common with virtually no never users in Westernized societies.
- Microbes could act as drugs, produce drugs, be a target for drug use, or be used as vehicles or adjuvants for drugs.
- Pharmacomicrobiomics studies the effect of the microbiome on drug metabolism and action; the microbiome composition and function are also influenced by drug intake.
- Prescribed drug use, particularly antibiotics and proton pump inhibitors, may affect gut microbiota diversity, especially when used over a longer period of time or during a critical time window.
- Large cohorts with valid prospectively collected and complete information on drug intake are needed to assess association with the microbiome or long-term outcomes.

INTRODUCTION

Our microbiome affects health and disease although the exact mechanisms are not entirely understood.[1–5] The microbiome is usually defined as the entire habitat, including the microorganisms (including bacteria, viruses, archaea, and fungi), their genetic material or genome, and the surrounding environmental conditions; the term microbiota refers to the assemblage of microorganisms present in a defined environment, such as the colon, vagina, or skin.[2] Beside the microbiome, many other factors affect our health, and (prescribed) drug use may be an important yet easily underestimated factor that potentially affects the whole body homeostasis.[6]

Drug use is extremely common, and it is well-known that there are differences in the effects and toxicity of drugs between individuals that may be partially attributable to the (gut) microbiome.[7,8] In addition, drug exposure could unintentionally alter the microbiome, although the extent and (long-term) consequences are only recently being investigated. Microbiome studies could also be confounded by drug use when

[a] Centre for Translational Microbiome Research, Department of Microbiology, Tumor and Cell Biology, Karolinska Institutet, Visionsgatan 4, Stockholm 17177, Sweden; [b] Science for Life Laboratory, Tomtebodavägen 23a, Stockholm 171 65, Sweden
* CTMR, Karolinska Institutet, Visionsgatan 4 South East- 171 64 Stockholm (Solna), Sweden.
E-mail address: nele.brusselaers@ki.se

Gastroenterol Clin N Am 48 (2019) 331–342
https://doi.org/10.1016/j.gtc.2019.04.002
0889-8553/19/© 2019 Elsevier Inc. All rights reserved.

evaluating microbiota compositions, or interactions may occur.[9] Ultimately, the microbiome has become a target for drug treatment, aiming for a shift from an unhealthy, dysbiotic state to a healthy microbiome, basically by using microbes as a drug (fecal stool transplants, probiotics) to reestablish or improve health.[10,11] Therefore, because the ample use of prescribed drugs and the increased interest microbiome research, the aim of this article is to address how drug use can affect the microbiome, and vice versa, and why assessing drug use in microbiome studies is important and challenging.

HOW COMMON IS PRESCRIBED DRUG USE?

Humans are exposed to (prescribed) drugs regularly during life, including vaccinations, painkillers, antibiotics, and contraceptives, not even thinking about antibiotic residuals ingested through food and drinking water. Statistics on prevalence of nonabusive prescribed drug use are sparse. In the United States, 47% of the total population had taken at least 1 prescription drug during the past 30-day window (study period 2011–2014), 52% of women and 43% of men; and 22% of children under 18 years of age.[12] In Sweden, 59% of all men and 74% of all women (66% combined) use prescribed drugs each year.[13] For children under 10 years of age and the elderly, 40% and 100%, respectively, do use prescribed drugs annually (based on all outpatient prescriptions during 2017; **Fig. 1**A).[13] In Sweden, medical practitioners have a relatively restrictive approach to drug use, in particular toward antibiotics, but still 20% of the total population uses outpatient (ambulatory) antibiotics every year (**Fig. 1**B, C), and up to 35% of those under 5 years old.[13] Some of the most commonly prescribed drugs are used by approximately 10% of the total population on an annual basis, including antidepressants, proton pump inhibitors (PPIs), beta-blockers, nonsteroidal antiinflammatory drugs, and statins (see **Fig 1**C).

There are several periods in life that may be critical considering the establishment and maintenance of a healthy microbiome, including childhood (in particular first 2 years of life),[7] and pregnancy (establishment of microbiome of the offspring)[14,15]; therefore, drug use during these periods may have long-term effects on the microbiota composition. Although drug use is restricted during pregnancy because of potential teratogenic effects, 27% to 93% of pregnant women fill at least 1 prescription, excluding vitamins and minerals.[16] The elderly age is also of particular interest considering drug–microbiome interactions; although the composition of the microbiome might be considered relatively stable, polypharmacy (≥5 drugs taken concomitantly) is frequent and coadministered drugs may have a different effect on the microbiome.[17,18] Of note, polypharmacy is present in 50% of individuals residing in European nursing homes, with extreme polypharmacy (>10 drugs) in 24%.[17,18]

PHARMACOMICROBIOMICS

Pharmacomicrobiomics is the term describing the interaction between the microbiome and drugs.[19–21] This term encompasses the study of how the microbiome compositional variance and functional variations affect drug disposition and response,[20,21] yet drugs also affect the microbiome. In addition, microbes could act as drugs (eg, stool transplants, probiotics), produce drugs (eg, digestive enzymes), and be a target for drug use (eg, antibiotics) or used as vehicles or adjuvants for drug delivery and vaccines.[21] Although the scientific interest in pharmacomicrobiomics only started booming with the recent advancements in microbiome research, drug metabolism by gut bacteria was already described half a century ago, and direct bacterial changes have been documented for an increasing number of drugs.[22–24] In the field of drug development and personalized medicine pharmacomicrobiomics may help to understand differences in treatment effects and interindividual heterogeneity.[25–27]

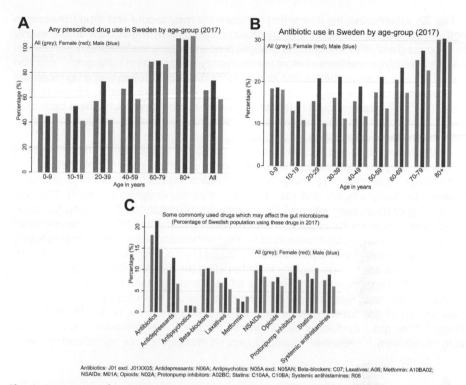

Antibiotics: J01 excl. J01XX05; Antidepressants: N06A; Antipsychotics: N05A excl. N05AN; Beta-blockers: C07; Laxatives: A06; Metformin: A10BA02; NSAIDs: M01A; Opioids: N02A; Protonpump inhibitors: A02BC; Statins: C10AA, C10BA; Systemic antihistamines: R06

Fig. 1. Frequency of prescribed drug use in Sweden in 2017. Proportion (%) of dispensed and prescribed drug use (excluding in-hospital and over-the-counter use) among Swedish residents during 2017 (*A*) at least 1 drug, categorized by age and sex, (*B*) at least 1 antibiotics categorized by age and sex, and (*C*) at least one commonly prescribed drug which may be affecting the gut microbiome, categorized by sex. (*Data from* Socialstyrelsen Statistics Database. Available at: https://www.socialstyrelsen.se/statistik/statistikdatabas/lakemedel.)

With 10^{10} to 10^{12} microbes per gram of luminal content, the colon has the highest concentration of bacteria along the gut (compared with 10^1–10^4 in the stomach); therefore, complex drug–microbial interactions are expected to mainly occur in the colon.[27] However, pharmacomicrobiomics is relevant not only to the gut microbiome. The effects of the vaginal microbiome, for instance, are also increasingly explored (eg, in human immunodeficiency virus treatment), and intratumoral bacteria may affect anticancer drugs.[7,19,25,26] In How can the microbiome affect drug metabolism?, the interactions between the microbiome and drug metabolism and vice versa are discussed in greater detail.

HOW CAN THE MICROBIOME AFFECT DRUG METABOLISM?

Microbiota-mediated alterations in drug metabolism may have an effect on the efficacy and toxicity of drugs, and also influence or induce drug–drug interactions.[7,8] The extent of the effect of the microbiome on drug metabolism depends largely on the type of drug, combination of drugs and genetics of the individual. Nonresponse for commonly prescribed drugs may be as high as 25% to 50%, and genetic factors only explain 20% to 95% of the variability in response to individual drugs.[27–29]

Fig. 2A schematizes the interaction between the microbiome and drug metabolism and action. On the one hand, the microbiome can directly metabolize drugs, mainly by producing enzymes with variable catalytic properties (biotransformation), with reduction and hydrolysis reactions as most common enzymatic reaction in the gut.[7,17,27,30] On the other hand, the microbiome can also produce drugs competing with drug receptors or indirectly influence the metabolizing capacity or immune system of the human host.[7,17,27,30] These biological activities led by the microbiome could affect both drug metabolism (pharmacokinetics) and action (pharmacodynamics), through the activation, potentiation, competition, or biodegradation of drug compounds.[17,19,27,30–32]

As discussed, drug-metabolizing enzymes produced by microbiota may activate or inactivate drugs or their metabolites, depending on which species are present.[17,30] For example, microbiome-related prodrug activation has been described for aminosalicylates (reducing efficacy and toxicity) and anthranoid laxatives including *Aloe vera* (increasing or decreasing efficacy). Drug inactivation related to microbiome has been described for digoxin (decreasing oral bioavailability), whereas microbiome-mediated drug deconjugation has been described for the chemotherapeutic irinotecan (increasing toxicity), and nonsteroidal antiinflammatory drugs (contributing to toxic mucosal damage).[30,33] There are several ongoing trials targeting the gut microbiota by probiotics or fecal microbial transplants to improve the efficacy and decrease the toxicity of drugs.[7]

Microbiome–drug reactions are not restricted to drugs reaching the colon. Even the microbiome of the small intestine may be responsible for the biotransformation of drugs.[33] The gut microbiome can indirectly influence liver functions, including bile acid metabolism.[17,34] Further, microbial-derived metabolites may mimic and compete

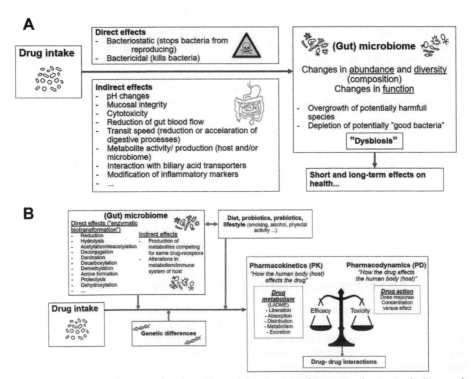

Fig. 2. Proposed mechanisms for the effect of (*A*) the microbiome on drug metabolism and action, and (*B*) drugs on the microbiome composition and function.

with drug intermediates of hepatic metabolic reactions, consequently inhibiting the metabolism of drugs such as paracetamol, potentially increasing the risk of hepato-toxicity.[17] The expression of hepatic enzymes or genes responsible for host meta-bolism may also be altered by the gut microbiome.[17] Drug metabolism may also be affected at other locations of the body, particularly if applied locally. *Gardnerella vaginalis* can, for example, biotransform vaginally delivered drugs such as the retroviral tenofovir, even before the host can turn it into the pharmaceutically active form, consequently reducing efficacy.[7,26]

HOW COULD PRESCRIBED DRUG USE AFFECT THE MICROBIOME?

Drug use may result in (un)intentional changes of the microbiome, which may be bene-ficial or detrimental to the host.[17] Some of the potential mechanisms are set forth in **Fig. 2**B. There could be direct bacteriostatic or bactericidal effects, also by drugs other than antibiotics, for example, antipsychotics.[35] The indirect effects may arise from pH changes, transit speed (including delayed gastric emptying), changes in the mucosal integrity, and others.[32,35] The stomach environment is highly acidic, and the pH in-creases gradually when passing through the gastrointestinal tract, ending up with a neutral pH in the colon.[36] Changes in the gastric pH, for example, by administering PPIs, may therefore result in changes of the gastric microbiota composition, and poten-tially even introduce changes further down the digestive track. Yet, the changes in the gut microbiome caused by PPIs are believed to be through pH-independent mecha-nisms because of the acid suppression in the proximal duodenum.[35]

So, drug use can change the composition of the microbiome in terms of abundance and diversity, and also change the function of the microbiome. When these changes cause a deviation from the normal microbiome, this is called dysbiosis. The normal or healthy state is not yet exactly determined for all microbiome locations, and may be depending on several characteristics such as age, sex, diet, and lifestyle.[37] To note, the disease states for which the drugs are administered may also cause microbiome changes that may be difficult to distinguish from the drug effects.[26] Drug-mediated al-terations of the microbiome may be transient, or have a long-term effect on the micro-biota composition. Because of the potential long-term changes, harmful or protective drug-induced microbiome alterations may even play a role in the development of can-cer or other diseases. For example, when *Helicobacter pylori* eradication therapy is administered successfully, this bacterium should be eliminated, contributing to a decreased risk of gastric cancer.[38] It has been described that tumor genesis is driven by microbial pathogens in 15% to 20% of cancer cases, but several species are described as having cancer protective effects, and the gut microbiome may affect response to cancer treatment.[39–41] For long-term drug-mediated changes of the microbiome affecting health, there is emerging population-based evidence on antibiotics, PPIs, metformin, and other agents, which may have practical implications in understanding cancer etiology and developing preventive approaches (chemopre-vention).[42–45] Also in the field of women's health, there is increasing evidence support-ing an association between drug use, the microbiome, and adverse events. It has, for example, been suggested that maternal PPI use during pregnancy may be affecting the risk of asthma and allergies in the offspring.[46] Because the microbiome may also play an important role in preterm birth and other pregnancy-related adverse events,[47,48] the safety and long-term effects of drugs affecting the microbiome may need further exploration for use during pregnancy.

Interestingly, drugs often contain substances without known pharmacologic properties. Excipients are defined as pharmacologically inert substances or nonactive ingredients, which are usually not absorbed from the gut, yet some may mediate micro-biome changes and alter composition or function.[17] Fermentable polysaccharide-based formulations (eg, used for delivery of probiotics and sulfasalazine) may, for example, promote the growth of certain species, and the polymer polyethylene glycol may change transit time in the gastrointestinal tract.[17] Potential excipient-induced microbiota changes may be difficult to distinguish from drug-induced changes,[17] and excipient effects should be considered when administering placebo products.

WHICH PRESCRIBED DRUGS AFFECT THE HUMAN MICROBIOME?

The effects of antibiotics on the gut microbiome are probably the most recognized and established, and have been investigated since the 1940s.[27,49] Until rather recently, most evidence was based on single cultivated strains of pathogenic bacteria or on cultivated bacteria originating from antibiotic-exposed hosts.[49] Antibiotic-initiated al-terations of the gut microbiome, as an ecologically complex system, may also result in metabolic changes in the host, increasing the risk of weight gain and obesity, changing the immune response and increasing susceptibility to other infections owing to a loss of colonization resistance, for example, to *Clostridium difficile* or *Salmonella* infec-tions.[27,49] Studies investigating the gut microbiota after antibiotic exposure showed a lower diversity overall and a lesser abundance of several bacterial species.[49] At least some degree of recovery occurs in most individuals, yet there is interindividual hetero-geneity and different effects for specific antibiotic types, with clindamycin showing the longest-lasting changes of the gut microbiome composition.[49]

Several nonantibiotic drugs have also showed to affect the (gut) microbiota compo-sition. A large Dutch–Flemish, population-based study identified 69 clinical and questionnaire-based variables to be associated with the variation of the fecal micro-biome, with drug use explaining the greatest total variance (10% of interindividual vari-ation) and also showing interaction with other covariate–microbiome associations. This study identified 13 drug groups associated with community composition variation,[50] and 19 drug groups in the Dutch part of the cohort. These 2 studies report associations with commonly prescribed drugs for several diseases, including antibiotics, osmotic laxatives, inflammatory bowel disease medication, female hormones, benzodiazepines, antidepressants, PPIs, statins, and antihistamines.[50,51] On a population level, PPIs seem to have the greatest effect on gut microbiome variation in terms of decreasing di-versity, potentially even greater than antibiotics,[52] which is especially worrying because of their widespread use.[52–54] A recent systematic review of nonantibiotic prescription drugs inducing gut dysbiosis summarizes the evidence for different commonly pre-scribed drug groups (PPIs, metformin, nonsteroidal antiinflammatory drugs, opioids, statins, and antipsychotics), their effect on diversity, and which specific species are affected. The authors reported increases in Gammaproteobacteria in particular, and some proposed mechanisms such as changes in the integrity of the intestinal epithelial barrier.[35] Yet, too little is currently known on the effect of other commonly[35] and less commonly prescribed drugs and the microbiome of the gut and other body locations.

METHODOLOGIC CHALLENGES

There are several challenges considering pharmacoepidemiologic studies designed to assess the associations between drug use, the microbiome and and/or (long-term) outcomes in the host.[4,55–57] Both the microbiome and drug use can be seen as expo-sures and prognostic markers, as well as risk factors for different outcomes. The chal-lenges include information bias, selection bias, confounding, power and generalizability, and temporal variations (**Table 1**). The high-dimensional dynamic

Table 1
Some of the challenges of studies assessing associations between drug use, the microbiome and the human host

Challenge	What?	Specific for Drug Use	Specific for Microbiome Research
Information bias	How are exposure and outcome measured, defined, and/or categorized? Does this misclassification occur in all individuals in the study (nondifferential) or only in some (differential)?	Ideally collected prospectively to avoid recall bias, so before onset of outcome. Prescribed drug use only or also over-the-counter use? Compliance to prescriptions?	Ideally longitudinal sample collection, to see if cause or effect. Sampling, preservation and assessment methods may affect which microbiota are detected. Is it established what the "healthy" state is?
Selection bias	How are the study participants selected, including the control group(s) Are there any differences in accepting enrollment or drop-out based on exposure (cohort design) or outcome (case control)?	Ideally nationwide and population-based to be representative. Definition of use and nonuse of drugs (eg, current users, past users, minimal number of prescriptions or cumulative dose to be considered exposed?). Indication for use (prevention, severity of disease)?	Large cohorts are needed to take into account interpersonal variety. Or restrict to very homogenous population.
Confounding	Which other variables could affect the association studied: sex, age, comorbidities, diet, environment, and so on?	Confounding by indication?	Genetic, ethnic, sociodemographic, and geographic variability.
Power	Is the study large enough to find differences if there are any?	Large numbers are needed especially if subgroup analyses are needed (eg, subtype of drugs, duration or dosage of exposure) or long-term outcomes are studied	Large interindividual variety, difficult to do power calculations specific for microbiome.
Generalizability	Are the results generalizable to other populations?	Are drug use/ prescription practices the same in other countries?	Are the "healthy" and dysbiosis microbiome composition and function the same in other cohorts?
Temporality and variation over time	Did the exposure occur before the outcome (otherwise reverse causation)? Is there an important variation over time?	Is there a critical time window of exposure, or critical duration of exposure?	How long are potential microbiome changes expected to last? How stable is the microbiome composition over time?

nature and extensive interindividual variability of the microbiome present important challenges. Most important, powerful statistical comparisons are challenging owing to the large amount of taxa and taxa combinations that are detected in each sample, substantially more than the amount of samples being collected.[4,58,59] Valid and standardized collection methods are needed to adequately define drug use and the microbiome composition and function.[60] Specific for the microbiome, sampling, storage, and processing need to be standardized and homogenized to decrease the risk of bias.[4,61] Considering drug use, the effects of the drug should also be distinguished from the effects of the underlying indication to evaluate the effect of confounding by indication, and likewise, drug use should ideally be considered when assessing the association between diseases and the microbiome.[9,43,44] Preferably, nonusers are compared with users with the same indication who are not using any drug (if ethically possible), or another drug. Yet, it could occur that virtually all individuals with a certain indication use this drug (eg, PPIs) so there are basically no or very few never users with the same indication who never used this drug.[43,44,62] A potential solution is to assess different risk groups of patients using these drugs, because some drugs may be used for different indications, which may have a different risk on the outcome.[43,44] If this does not work, subgroup analyses by dosage, timing, and duration may shed some light, but usually these factors also correlate strongly with the severity of the disease.

A good study design is also needed to avoid selection bias and enable collection of high quality data on factors that may confound the association of interest, including demographics, ethnogeographic differences, diet, socioeconomic, environmental, and lifestyle factors.[63] Temporal variations in both drug use and microbiome compositions may also complicate analyses, and therefore larger samples sizes, prospectively ascertained study participants, and/or sequential testing may be considered to optimize analyses and interpretation.[36,64] To conclude, good planning and study design are crucial, because in particular the biases may not be correctable when data collection has started. This factor may imply large and representative cohorts with high-quality information on drug intake and validated and standardized methods to collect, store, and assess microbiome alterations. All studies do have limitations, which should be acknowledged and the potential impact on the interpretation of the findings should be assessed.

SUMMARY

Drug use is common, and microbiome research is booming, resulting in an increasing interest in the interplay between these entities and their combined effects on health and disease. The microbiome may affect the metabolism and action of drugs, leading to changes in efficacy and toxicity, and potential drug–drug interactions. The composition and function of microbiome may also be affected by drug use, potentially even showing long-term effects detectable on the population level. To make it more complex, microbiota can also be used as drugs, aiming for intentional changes of microbiome composition, for example, by using probiotics or stool transplants to restore a dysbiotic composition and improve the health of the individual. There are many challenges in this field, and more research will result in a better understanding of these complex mechanisms. In the field of pharmacology, this process may optimize drug development and personalized medicine. In the microbiome field, it is important to keep the importance of interpersonal variation in mind caused by drug use, and to distinguish the effects of the drugs and the underlying indications. In medical research in general, it may be important to consider the potential long-term effects of drugs on health through potential drug–microbiome interactions, which are currently insufficiently understood. Establishing causal relationships may be the penultimate goal of all research, to establish or improve treatments or prevention methods.[65] Yet, causality can never be established based on a single study.[62] Especially in the microbiome field, multidisciplinary endeavors and different study designs seem crucial, going from basic science laboratory and animal experiments, to translational clinical research and pure epidemiologic studies, including studies based on nation-wide prospective drug registries, to generate and test hypotheses.

REFERENCES

1. Blum HE. The human microbiome. Adv Med Sci 2017;62(2):414–20.
2. Marchesi JR, Ravel J. The vocabulary of microbiome research: a proposal. Microbiome 2015;3:31.
3. Smith MI, Turpin W, Tyler AD, et al. Microbiome analysis - from technical advances to biological relevance. F1000prime Rep 2014;6:51.
4. Tyler AD, Smith MI, Silverberg MS. Analyzing the human microbiome: a "how to" guide for physicians. Am J Gastroenterol 2014;109(7):983–93.
5. Gilbert JA, Blaser MJ, Caporaso JG, et al. Current understanding of the human microbiome. Nat Med 2018;24(4):392–400.
6. Gupta VK, Paul S, Dutta C. Geography, ethnicity or subsistence-specific variations in human microbiome composition and diversity. Front Microbiol 2017;8:1162.
7. Wilkinson EM, Ilhan ZE, Herbst-Kralovetz MM. Microbiota-drug interactions: impact on metabolism and efficacy of therapeutics. Maturitas 2018;112:53–63.
8. Noh K, Kang YR, Nepal MR, et al. Impact of gut microbiota on drug metabolism: an update for safe and effective use of drugs. Arch Pharm Res 2017;40(12):1345–55.
9. Devkota S. MICROBIOME. Prescription drugs obscure microbiome analyses. Science 2016;351(6272):452–3.
10. Tsai YL, Lin TL, Chang CJ, et al. Probiotics, prebiotics and amelioration of diseases. J Biomed Sci 2019;26(1):3.
11. Kelly CR, Kahn S, Kashyap P, et al. Update on fecal microbiota transplantation 2015: indications, methodologies, mechanisms, and outlook. Gastroenterology 2015;149(1):223–37.
12. Centre for Disease Control and Prevention. Trend Tables: prescription drug use in the past 30 days, by sex, race and Hispanic origin and age 2016. Available at: https://www.cdc.gov/nchs/data/hus/2016/079.pdf. Accessed January 1, 2019.
13. The Swedish Board of Health and Welfare (Socialstyrelsen) - Statistical Database. Available at: http://www.socialstyrelsen.se/statistik/statistikdatabas. Accessed December 1, 2018.
14. Neu J. The microbiome during pregnancy and early postnatal life. Semin Fetal Neonatal Med 2016;21(6):373–9.
15. Blaser MJ, Dominguez-Bello MG. The human microbiome before birth. Cell Host Microbe 2016;20(5):558–60.
16. Daw JR, Hanley GE, Greyson DL, et al. Prescription drug use during pregnancy in developed countries: a systematic review. Pharmacoepidemiol Drug Saf 2011;20(9):895–902.
17. Walsh J, Griffin BT, Clarke G, et al. Drug-gut microbiota interactions: implications for neuropharmacology. Br J Pharmacol 2018;175(24):4415–29.

59. Tsilimigras MC, Fodor AA. Compositional data analysis of the microbiome: fundamentals, tools, and challenges. Ann Epidemiol 2016;26(5):330–5.
60. Sinha R, Chen J, Amir A, et al. Collecting fecal samples for microbiome analyses in epidemiology studies. Cancer Epidemiol Biomarkers Prev 2016;25(2):407–16.
61. Fu BC, Randolph TW, Lim U, et al. Characterization of the gut microbiome in epidemiologic studies: the multiethnic cohort experience. Ann Epidemiol 2016; 26(5):373–9.
62. Brusselaers N, Engstrand L, Lagergren J. PPI use and oesophageal cancer: what if the results are true? Cancer Epidemiol 2018;54:139–40.
63. Singh P, Manning SD. Impact of age and sex on the composition and abundance of the intestinal microbiota in individuals with and without enteric infections. Ann Epidemiol 2016;26(5):380–5.
64. Hanson BM, Weinstock GM. The importance of the microbiome in epidemiologic research. Ann Epidemiol 2016;26(5):301–5.
65. Mai V, Prosperi M, Yaghjyan L. Moving microbiota research toward establishing causal associations that represent viable targets for effective public health interventions. Ann Epidemiol 2016;26(5):306–10.

Gut-Brain Interactions

Implications for a Role of the Gut Microbiota in the Treatment and Prognosis of Anorexia Nervosa and Comparison to Type I Diabetes

Daria Igudesman, MS[a], Megan Sweeney, MPH, RD[a],
Ian M. Carroll, PhD[a], Elizabeth J. Mayer-Davis, PhD[a],
Cynthia M. Bulik, PhD[a,b,c],*

KEYWORDS

- Anorexia nervosa • Diabetes • Microbiome • Microbiota • Metabolism

KEY POINTS

- Anorexia nervosa is highly refractory, and novel treatments are needed to improve prognosis.
- The gut microbiota is dysregulated in anorexia nervosa and may be a new avenue for research in reducing discomfort during refeeding.
- Metabolism often is dysregulated in anorexia nervosa and type 1 diabetes (T1D), which share common genetic alterations, disordered eating patterns, and features of gut microbial dysbiosis.

Disclosure Statement: Dr D. Igudesman receives funding from 1UC4DK101132-01. Dr I. Carroll is a Consultant for Vivilex and former consultant for Salix Pharmaceuticals and receives funding from National Institutes of Health (NIH) (R21-AI125800-01-02); National Institute of Mental Health (NIMH) (R01-MH105684-03) and Arthritis Foundation (A17-1004-001). Dr E. Mayer-Davis receives funding from NIH (1UC4DK101132-01; 2R01DK077949-4; 1UC4DK108173-03; 2P30DK056350-16; 1DP3DK113358-02; and R01DK115434-02), Centers for Disease Control and Prevention (CDC) (1U18DP006138-03), and Helmsley. Dr C.M. Bulik is an author and royalty recipient from Pearson and Walker and grant recipient and Scientific Advisory Board member for Shire and receives funding from Swedish Research Council (Vetenskapsrådet Dnr: 538-2013-8864) and NIH (R01, MN105684-03, Principal Investigator, Carroll). Dr M. Sweeney has nothing to disclose.
[a] Department of Nutrition, University of North Carolina at Chapel Hill, 135 Dauer Drive, Chapel Hill, NC 27599, USA; [b] Department of Psychiatry, University of North Carolina at Chapel Hill, 101 Manning Drive, Chapel Hill, NC 27599, USA; [c] Department of Medical Epidemiology and Biostatistics, Karolinska Institutet, Stockholm, Sweden
* Corresponding author.
E-mail address: cbulik@med.unc.edu

food. Increased colonic permeability and altered tight junction protein expression have been demonstrated in activity-based anorexia mice.[44] Higher levels of mucin-degrading *Akkermansia muciniphila* also have been observed in athletes. The investigators speculated that *A. muciniphila* may improve barrier function by mechanisms still not fully understood, whereas others hypothesized that increased levels of the microbe would compromise the mucus layer of the epithelium and thereby the integrity of the intestinal barrier.[58,59]

Studies of forced activity in rodents could reveal how excessive exercise could affect the gut microbiota in AN, because it may better approximate the compulsive, compensatory exercise associated with AN rather than voluntary exercise. For example, Allen and colleagues[60] found that mice subjected to forced treadmill running had greater microbial diversity and altered gut microbial composition relative to mice exposed to voluntary wheel running. Although increased gut microbial diversity generally is associated with better health, here it was related to an expansion of rare bacterial species. The forced treadmill running mouse feces also exhibited a predominance of taxa that have been linked to disease states.

SHORT-CHAIN FATTY ACIDS
Role in Human Health

SCFAs—dietary metabolites produced by gut microbial fermentation of indigestible dietary carbohydrates—are an emerging topic of interest in metabolic health and weight management. Butyrate is a widely studied SCFA that is known to stimulate goblet cell mucin synthesis, which promotes gut health by lubricating and protecting epithelial cells. Butyrate also serves as a salient energy source for the intestinal epithelium.[61] Butyrate is primarily found in milk fat.[62] SCFA production could be reduced in AN due to avoidance of fat-containing food products (13% of calories consumed from fat have been noted in AN patients vs 31% in controls).[63]

Fecal Short-Chain Fatty Acids are Reduced in Anorexia Nervosa

Most studies have reported reduced fecal SCFAs in AN patients compared with controls. Borgo and colleagues[32] detected significantly lower fecal concentrations of total SCFAs ($P = .041$), butyrate ($P = .045$), and propionate ($P = .028$); notably, their finding of decreased butyrate is consistent with decreased carbohydrate-fermenting genera *Ruminococcus* ($P = .019$), *Roseburia* ($P = .037$), and *Clostridium* ($P = .031$). Decreased acetate ($P = .0003$) and propionate ($P = .001$) were found in AN patients in Japan compared with healthy controls.[64] By contrast, Mack and colleagues[25] reported comparable fecal concentrations of total SCFAs, acetate, butyrate, and propionate in AN patients and controls. They nevertheless detected reduced butyrate as a percentage of total SCFAs among AN patients on admission, compared with discharge and with NW controls, which concurred with a reduced abundance of butyrate-producing *Roseburia*. Furthermore, butyrate concentration correlated with *Roseburia* abundance in all 3 groups. The inconsistencies across studies may reflect compositional differences that occur across geographic regions.[65,66]

To remedy reduced SCFA production in AN patients, some investigators have proposed administering butyrate-producing *Roseburia* or supplementing directly with SCFAs.[25,67] Theoretically, increased intake of carbohydrates and prebiotic fibers also would enhance SCFA production. The bacterial fermentation of carbohydrates, however, also would contribute to gas, bloating, and distention, producing physical discomfort after meals and potentially exacerbating body image concerns.

PARALLELS BETWEEN ANOREXIA NERVOSA AND TYPE 1 DIABETES
Energy Dysregulation

Alterations in energy metabolism are central to both type 1 diabetes (T1D) and AN. Similar to the catabolic state that occurs due to starvation in AN,[68] severe weight loss is a feature of untreated T1D.[68,69] Even when treated, elevated resting energy expenditure occurs in individuals with T1D relative to prediction equations for healthy individuals.[70,71] Although reduced resting energy expenditure occurs in underweight AN,[72] many patients experience hypermetabolism during refeeding for unknown reasons.[73]

Etiology, Prevalence, and Complications of Disordered Eating in Type 1 Diabetes

It is tempting to speculate that the increased prevalence of disordered eating among individuals with T1D is a function of constant carbohydrate counting for blood glucose control and intense attention to weight. Although this behavior is initially medically driven, food restriction, defined as restraint, or self-imposed resistance to food consumption,[74] is associated with undesirable shifts in behavior and metabolism. One such behavior includes insulin restriction,[75] which can lead to uncontrolled blood glucose[76,77] and thus acute and chronic health complications. Schober and colleagues[78] found that reasons most commonly reported for insulin omission included denial of the disease in situations with peers (30%), self-destructive behavior and suicidal ideation (28%), fear of severe hypoglycemia (24%), and intention to lose weight (15.5.%). Conversely, intentional insulin overdosing to enable binge eating also has been commonly reported among individuals with T1D.[78] Elevated BMI also may result, because restraint can lead to uncontrolled overeating when individuals cease to limit their food intake.[79,80]

Furthermore, co-occurring T1D and ED may interact to synergistically worsen health outcomes. In 1 study, mortality via diabetes-related metabolic complications was increased with co-occurring T1D and AN, compared with either disorder alone (standardized mortality ratio 4.06, 8.86, and 14.5 for T1D, AN, and T1D and AN combined, respectively).[81] Peveler and colleagues[77] reported that among individuals with T1D, those with EDs had a higher baseline hemoglobin A_{1c} (HbA$_{1c}$), a 3-month measure of blood glucose, than those without an ED (11.9 vs 9.4, $P = .009$). HbA$_{1c}$ was not associated, however, with ED status at 8-year to 12-year follow-up points, suggesting that in some instances, disordered eating behaviors may normalize after adolescence.[77]

A systematic review suggests that both BN and the combined presence of BN and AN are significantly elevated in patients with T1D compared with controls (both $P<.05$).[82] Of 550 female patients with T1D, 1% had lifetime AN and 16.2% had lifetime BN.[83] Subthreshold disordered eating also is prevalent, with 1 study reporting a greater proportion of girls ages 9 to 14 with T1D reporting 2 or more unhealthy eating behaviors compared with nondiabetic controls ($P<.0005$).[84]

Gut Microbial Dysbiosis in Type 1 Diabetes

Although shifts in dietary behaviors rapidly and reliably alter the enteric microbial community, much of the literature linking T1D with changes in the gut microbiota has focused on infants and children proximal to T1D onset. Most[26,27] but not all[85] studies report reduced enteric microbial diversity among patients who develop autoimmunity to pancreatic islet cells compared with controls. Compositional differences were reported in 2 independent cohorts of Mexican and Finnish children displaying increased *Bacteroides* among T1D cases and *Prevotella* among controls.[86,87] Another research team found that 2 species from the *Bacteroides* genus were significantly increased among Finnish T1D case children months before diabetes onset.[88] Yet other studies reported reduced abundance of *Bifidobacterium* in patients compared with controls,[89,90] although other compositional differences have been less consistently observed.[26,85,89]

Similar to AN, reduced fecal SCFAs have been observed among individuals with T1D compared with controls. Despite a trend toward increased fiber consumption among individuals with T1D compared with nondiabetic controls in 1 study, control participants had increased levels of plasma acetate and propionate compared with the T1D group, although total fecal SCFAs were similar.[91] This may suggest enhanced utilization of SCFA metabolites by individuals with T1D before they reach the plasma, perhaps to fulfill functions related to gut epithelial integrity.

The Gut Microbiota is Associated with Weight Status and Glycemia

Gut microbial composition also has been found to shift reliably in association with changes in weight status and metabolic parameters—including glucose homeostasis—in both animal and human models, which is relevant considering the increased prevalence of overweight and obesity among individuals with T1D.[92] For instance, Rabot and colleagues[93] showed that germ-free mice fed a high-fat diet were able to maintain euglycemia (normal blood glucose), although conventionally raised mice with gut microbiota that had been allowed to colonize naturally, developed glucose intolerance, and had higher plasma insulin concentrations in both a fed and 6-hour unfed state. In a study with human participants, Nadal and colleagues[94] found that changes in blood glucose significantly correlated with changes in proportions of gut microbial groups in adolescents participating in a weight loss intervention, regardless of weight loss outcome ($P = .006$). Diagnostic crossover is common in EDs, meaning that during the course of individuals' illness, they may transition across diagnostic presentations (AN, BN, and BED),[95] which can entail considerable fluctuations in weight. No work has yet been done to understand how the gut microbiota may be implicated in these longitudinal changes in symptom presentation.

Genetics

The association between AN and T1D may reflect shared genetic variants, including those related to metabolism. An AN GWAS detected 1 genome-wide significant variant for AN,[8] which previously was found associated with T1D. Significant genetic correlations emerged between AN and multiple metabolic traits implicated in T1D, including insulin resistance, fasting insulin, fasting glucose, and cholesterol and lipid measures.[8] These findings are consistent with evidence of increased ED prevalence and disordered eating among individuals with T1D as well as increased risk of autoimmune disorders, especially of endocrinological and gastroenterological types, among individuals with ED.[47] Considerably more work is essential to confirm and dissect the nature of this relationship. Larger sample sizes for AN GWAS are critical first steps for any more detailed analysis of the association.

FUTURE DIRECTIONS

It is vital to consider genetic, metabolic, and psychological factors that influence AN and multifactorial disorders, such as T1D, in which symptoms of disordered eating, energy dysregulation, and gut microbial dysbiosis manifest. Fecal microbiota transplantation (FMT), or the transfer of fecal microbiota from healthy donors to diseased patients, is 1 potential treatment that is on the horizon for many disease states, including T1D and AN,[96] based on its effectiveness at treating *Clostridium difficile* infections.[97] One challenge with respect to translational application of FMT to other disease states is donor screening, because systematic assessments of donor health have yet to be established. Furthermore, no standard exists for ideal gut microbial composition, although screening out individuals with pathogenic gut microorganisms is critical. Preliminary evidence exists, however, that FMT can improve metabolic phenotypes, including median rate of glucose disappearance and insulin sensitivity among male patients with metabolic syndrome ($P<.05$), which is relevant in light of obesity-associated insulin resistance that can develop in T1D.[98,99] Thus, experimenting with FMT and other adjunct therapies in treating symptoms of AN and T1D may provide insight into how the gut microbiota contribute to disease pathology and prognosis.

SUMMARY

Through their effects on the intestinal epithelium and immunity, gut microbes and their fermentative byproducts can influence metabolic and psychological health parameters in patients with AN. Integrative therapies that restore gut microbial health also may benefit individuals with conditions in which gut microbial dysbiosis manifests, as in T1D, because individuals in this population experience difficulties with weight stabilization and altered metabolic traits and are vulnerable to developing symptoms of disordered eating.

Although the clinical implications of the brain-gut-microbiota axis are not yet fully understood in AN, targeted probiotics and antibiotics represent 2 mechanisms by which augmenting the gut microbiota can serve as an ancillary therapy for lessening severity of bloating and discomfort during treatment. Specifically, antibiotics could be used to eliminate known pathogens that disrupt intestinal integrity, whereas targeted probiotics may help to restore beneficial species known to promote gut epithelial health. Thus, the authors conclude that controlled studies investigating use of such novel therapies, including FMT, should be undertaken as part of an interdisciplinary approach to address metabolic and psychological factors that influence acute and long-term health outcomes in AN and T1D. The authors highlight again that work on the role of the intestinal microbiota in EDs is both limited and confined to AN. As is commonly the case, biological research in EDs starts with AN before progressing to the other EDs presentations. Yet, in many ways, EDs are model conditions on in which to explore the gut-brain axis given the centrality of eating and metabolic factors to the illnesses. The authors encourage investigators to expand on this early work by conducting studies on the other EDs (both in youth and adults) to develop a more comprehensive picture of the role that the intestinal microbiota plays in the development and maintenance of and recovery from these debilitating illnesses.

REFERENCES

1. Galmiche M, Déchelotte P, Lambert G, et al. Prevalence of eating disorders over the 2000–2018 period: a systematic literature review. Am J of Clin Nutr 2019;109: 1402–13.
2. Keski-Rahkonen A, Mustelin L. Epidemiology of eating disorders in Europe: prevalence, incidence, comorbidity, course, consequences, and risk factors. Curr Opin Psychiatry 2016;29:340–5.
3. Nakai Y, Fukushima M, Taniguchi A, et al. Comparison of DSM-IV versus proposed DSM-5 diagnostic criteria for eating disorders in a Japanese sample. Eur Eat Disord Rev 2013;21:8–14.

4. Keel PK, Brown TA, Holm-Denoma J, et al. Comparison of DSM-IV versus proposed DSM-5 diagnostic criteria for eating disorders: reduction of eating disorder not otherwise specified and validity. Int J Eat Disord 2011;44:553–60.

5. Machado PP, Goncalves S, Hoek HW. DSM-5 reduces the proportion of EDNOS cases: evidence from community samples. Int J Eat Disord 2013;46:60–5.

6. Schaumberg K, Welch E, Breithaupt L, et al. The science behind the Academy for Eating Disorders' nine truths about eating disorders. Eur Eat Disord Rev 2017;25: 432–50.

7. Yilmaz Z, Hardaway JA, Bulik CM. Genetics and epigenetics of eating disorders. Adv Genomics Genet 2015;5:131–50.

8. Duncan L, Yilmaz Z, Gaspar H, et al. Significant locus and metabolic genetic correlations revealed in genome-wide association study of anorexia nervosa. Am J Psychiatry 2017;174:850–8.

9. Treasure J, Zipfel S, Micali N, et al. Anorexia nervosa. Nat Rev Dis Primers 2015; 1:15074.

10. Zipfel S, Giel KE, Bulik CM, et al. Anorexia nervosa: aetiology, assessment, and treatment. Lancet Psychiatry 2015;2:1099–111.

11. Strober M, Freeman R, Morrell W. The long-term course of severe anorexia nervosa in adolescents: survival analysis of recovery, relapse, and outcome predictors over 10–15 years in a prospective study. Int J Eat Disord 1997;22:339–60.

12. Lock J, Le Grange D, Agras WS, et al. Randomized clinical trial comparing family-based treatment with adolescent-focused individual therapy for adolescents with anorexia nervosa. Arch Gen Psychiatry 2010;67:1025–32.

13. Eisler I, Simic M, Russell GF, et al. A randomised controlled treatment trial of two forms of family therapy in adolescent anorexia nervosa: a five-year follow-up. J Child Psychol Psychiatry 2007;48:552–60.

14. Keski-Rahkonen A, Hoek HW, Susser ES, et al. Epidemiology and course of anorexia nervosa in the community. Am J Psychiatry 2007;164:1259–65.

15. Watson H, Bulik C. Update on the treatment of anorexia nervosa: review of clinical trials, practice guidelines and emerging interventions. Psychol Med 2013;43: 2477–500.

16. Arcelus J, Mitchell AJ, Wales J, et al. Mortality rates in patients with anorexia nervosa and other eating disorders: a meta-analysis of 36 studies. Arch Gen Psychiatry 2011;68:724–31.

17. Pompili M, Mancinelli I, Girardi P, et al. Suicide in anorexia nervosa: a meta-analysis. Int J Eat Disord 2004;36:99–103.

18. Zipfel S, Löwe B, Reas DL, et al. Long-term prognosis in anorexia nervosa: lessons from a 21-year follow-up study. Lancet 2000;355:721–2.

19. Pariante CM, Lightman SL. The HPA axis in major depression: classical theories and new developments. Trends Neurosci 2008;31:464–8.

20. Mayer EA. Gut feelings: the emerging biology of gut–brain communication. Nat Rev Neurosci 2011;12:453.

21. O'Mahony S, Clarke G, Borre Y, et al. Serotonin, tryptophan metabolism and the brain-gut-microbiome axis. Behav Brain Res 2015;277:32–48.

22. Rieder R, Wisniewski PJ, Alderman BL, et al. Microbes and mental health: a review. Brain Behav Immun 2017;66:9–17.

23. Sherwin E, Rea K, Dinan TG, et al. A gut (microbiome) feeling about the brain. Curr Opin Gastroenterol 2016;32:96–102.

24. van de Wouw M, Schellekens H, Dinan TG, et al. Microbiota-gut-brain axis: modulator of host metabolism and appetite. J Nutr 2017;147:727–45.

25. Mack I, Cuntz U, Grämer C, et al. Weight gain in anorexia nervosa does not ameliorate the faecal microbiota, branched chain fatty acid profiles, and gastrointestinal complaints. Sci Rep 2016;6:26752.
26. Giongo A, Gano KA, Crabb DB, et al. Toward defining the autoimmune microbiome for type 1 diabetes. ISME J 2011;5:82.
27. Kostic AD, Gevers D, Siljander H, et al. The dynamics of the human infant gut microbiome in development and in progression toward type 1 diabetes. Cell Host Microbe 2015;17:260–73.
28. Kleiman SC, Watson HJ, Bulik-Sullivan EC, et al. The intestinal microbiota in acute anorexia nervosa and during renourishment: relationship to depression, anxiety, and eating disorder psychopathology. Psychosom Med 2015;77:969.
29. Franko DL, Tabri N, Keshaviah A, et al. Predictors of long-term recovery in anorexia nervosa and bulimia nervosa: data from a 22-year longitudinal study. J Psychiatr Res 2018;96:183–8.
30. Glenny EM, Bulik-Sullivan EC, Tang Q, et al. Eating disorders and the intestinal microbiota: mechanisms of energy homeostasis and behavioral influence. Curr Psychiatry Rep 2017;19:51.
31. Armougom F, Henry M, Vialettes B, et al. Monitoring bacterial community of human gut microbiota reveals an increase in Lactobacillus in obese patients and Methanogens in anorexic patients. PLoS One 2009;4:e7125.
32. Borgo F, Riva A, Benetti A, et al. Microbiota in anorexia nervosa: the triangle between bacterial species, metabolites and psychological tests. PLoS One 2017; 12:e0179739.
33. Mathur R, Kim G, Morales W, et al. Intestinal Methanobrevibacter smithii but not total bacteria is related to diet-induced weight gain in rats. Obesity (Silver Spring) 2013;21:748–54.
34. Mbakwa CA, Penders J, Savelkoul PH, et al. Gut colonization with Methanobrevibacter smithii is associated with childhood weight development. Obesity (Silver Spring) 2015;23:2508–16.
35. Samuel BS, Gordon JI. A humanized gnotobiotic mouse model of host–archaeal–bacterial mutualism. Proc Natl Acad Sci U S A 2006;103:10011–6.
36. Basseri RJ, Basseri B, Pimentel M, et al. Intestinal methane production in obese individuals is associated with a higher body mass index. Gastroenterol Hepatol (N Y) 2012;8:22.
37. Mathur R, Amichai MM, Mirocha JM, et al. Concomitant methane and hydrogen production in humans is associated with a higher body mass index. Gastroenterology 2011;140:S-335.
38. Cummings JH. The large intestine in nutrition and disease. Belgium: Institut Danone Brussels, Belgium; 1997.
39. Kamal N, Chami T, Andersen A, et al. Delayed gastrointestinal transit times in anorexia nervosa and bulimia nervosa. Gastroenterology 1991;101:1320–4.
40. Vandeputte D, Falony G, Vieira-Silva S, et al. Stool consistency is strongly associated with gut microbiota richness and composition, enterotypes and bacterial growth rates. Gut 2015;65(1):57–62.
41. Mehler PS, Brown C. Anorexia nervosa–medical complications. J Eat Disord 2015;3:11.
42. Pimentel M, Lembo A, Chey WD, et al. Rifaximin therapy for patients with irritable bowel syndrome without constipation. N Engl J Med 2011;364:22–32.
43. Ringel-Kulka T, Palsson OS, Maier D, et al. Probiotic bacteria Lactobacillus acidophilus NCFM and Bifidobacterium lactis Bi-07 versus placebo for the

82. Mannucci E, Rotella F, Ricca V, et al. Eating disorders in patients with type 1 diabetes: a meta-analysis. J Endocrinol Invest 2005;28:417–9.
83. Birk R, Spencer ML. The prevalence of anorexia nervosa, bulimia, and induced glycosuria in IDDM females. Diabetes Educ 1989;15:336–41.
84. Colton P, Olmsted M, Daneman D, et al. Disturbed eating behavior and eating disorders in preteen and early teenage girls with type 1 diabetes: a case-controlled study. Diabetes Care 2004;27:1654–9.
85. Murri M, Leiva I, Gomez-Zumaquero JM, et al. Gut microbiota in children with type 1 diabetes differs from that in healthy children: a case-control study. BMC Med 2013;11:46.
86. Brown CT, Davis-Richardson AG, Giongo A, et al. Gut microbiome metagenomics analysis suggests a functional model for the development of autoimmunity for type 1 diabetes. PLoS One 2011;6:e25792.
87. Mejía-León ME, Petrosino JF, Ajami NJ, et al. Fecal microbiota imbalance in Mexican children with type 1 diabetes. Sci Rep 2014;4:3814.
88. Davis-Richardson AG, Ardissone AN, Dias R, et al. Bacteroides dorei dominates gut microbiome prior to autoimmunity in Finnish children at high risk for type 1 diabetes. Front Microbiol 2014;5:678.
89. de Goffau MC, Fuentes S, van den Bogert B, et al. Aberrant gut microbiota composition at the onset of type 1 diabetes in young children. Diabetologia 2014;57:1569–77.
90. Soyucen E, Gulcan A, Aktuglu-Zeybek AC, et al. Differences in the gut microbiota of healthy children and those with type 1 diabetes. Pediatr Int 2014;56:336–43.
91. De Groot PF, Belzer C, Aydin Ö, et al. Distinct fecal and oral microbiota composition in human type 1 diabetes, an observational study. PLoS One 2017;12: e0188475.
92. Kilpatrick ES, Rigby AS, Atkin SL. Insulin resistance, the metabolic syndrome, and complication risk in type 1 diabetes:"double diabetes" in the Diabetes Control and Complications Trial. Diabetes Care 2007;30:707–12.
93. Rabot S, Membrez M, Bruneau A, et al. Germ-free C57BL/6J mice are resistant to high-fat-diet-induced insulin resistance and have altered cholesterol metabolism. FASEB J 2010;24:4948–59.
94. Nadal I, Santacruz A, Marcos A, et al. Shifts in clostridia, bacteroides and immunoglobulin-coating fecal bacteria associated with weight loss in obese adolescents. Int J Obes (Lond) 2009;33:758–67.
95. Schaumberg K, Jangmo A, Thornton L, et al. Patterns of diagnostic flux in eating disorders: a longitudinal population study in Sweden. Psychol Med 2019;49(5): 819–27.
96. Borody TJ, Khoruts A. Fecal microbiota transplantation and emerging applications. Nat Rev Gastroenterol Hepatol 2012;9:88.
97. Brandt LJ, Aroniadis OC, Mellow M, et al. Long-term follow-up of colonoscopic fecal microbiota transplant for recurrent Clostridium difficile infection. Am J Gastroenterol 2012;107:1079.
98. Polsky S, Ellis SL. Obesity, insulin resistance, and type 1 diabetes mellitus. Curr Opin Endocrinol Diabetes Obes 2015;22:277–82.
99. Vrieze A, Van Nood E, Holleman F, et al. Transfer of intestinal microbiota from lean donors increases insulin sensitivity in individuals with metabolic syndrome. Gastroenterology 2012;143:913–6.e7.

The Development of the Human Microbiome

Why Moms Matter

Derrick M. Chu, PhD, Gregory C. Valentine, MD, MEd,
Maxim D. Seferovic, PhD, Kjersti M. Aagaard, MD, PhD*

KEYWORDS

• Microbiome • Mode of delivery • Development

KEY POINTS

• The intrauterine environment retains a low-abundance, low-biomass microbiome that may be important for establishing tolerance to commensal organisms in utero.
• Multiple perinatal factors beyond whether the infant was born via cesarean delivery show a lasting impact on the developing human microbiome.
• Prematurely delivered neonates are more likely to harbor pathobionts, which may explain why these neonates have higher rates of necrotizing enterocolitis and other conditions associated with prematurity. Whether these pathobionts are causally related to preterm labor and birth remains unknown.

INTRODUCTION

Bacteria and viruses, colloquially referred to as germs, have historically been regarded by the lay public as harmful to human health and thus avoidable at all costs, particularly during pregnancy. Hand sanitizer and antibacterial soaps are ubiquitous in homes and hospitals alike, whereas the media are rife with reports on the next antibiotic-resistant "superbug" and the looming threat of bioterrorism in the form of genetically modified microbes. However, it might frighten even the mildest of germophobes to know that the human body is cohabitated with trillions of commensal bacteria that are essential for our health. Current estimates indicate that the number of microbes that inhabit the entire body roughly equals the total number of cells that comprise the human body.[1] The bulk of this biomass is found in the large and small intestines, although bacteria are known to inhabit nearly every niche throughout the body, including the skin and the vagina.[2] Together, these bacteria comprise an individual's

Disclosure: The authors have nothing to disclose.
Department of Obstetrics & Gynecology, Division of Maternal-Fetal Medicine 1 Baylor Plaza, Houston, TX 77030, USA
* Corresponding author. Department of Obstetrics & Gynecology, Division of Maternal-Fetal Medicine, Baylor College of Medicine, Texas Children's Hospital, 1 Baylor Plaza, Houston,TX 77030, USA.
E-mail address: aagaardt@bcm.edu

Gastroenterol Clin N Am 48 (2019) 357–375
https://doi.org/10.1016/j.gtc.2019.04.004
gastro.theclinics.com

microbiota and encode for thousands of metabolic functions known in totality as the microbiome. The community genetic repertoire encoded by both human and microbe is referred to as the metagenome.

Before the microbiome can be attributed to disease risk and pathogenesis, normal acquisition and development of the microbiome must be well understood. For this reason, acquisition of the microbiome in the first few years of life has been intensely studied over the past decade and our laboratory has joined with others to pioneer these efforts. The historical paradigm assumes that neonates are born sterile and are colonized differently depending on mode of delivery (ie, cesarean vs vaginal).[3,4] However, emerging evidence showing both a low biomass and low abundance of microbes harbored in the uterine decidua and fallopian tubes, as well as in association with the amniotic fluid, placenta, amnion, and chorion, and the developing fetus has challenged this notion, indicating that exposure to microbes (or at least their metagenomes) may begin well before delivery.[5–29]

This article first explores the evidence surrounding in utero microbial exposures and the significance of this exposure in the proper development of the fetal and neonatal microbiome. It then delves into the development of the fetal and neonatal microbiome and its relationship to preterm birth, feeding practices (breast milk vs formula), and mode of delivery. In addition, it evaluates the impact of the maternal diet on the developing fetal and neonatal microbiome.

HOW PURE IS THE WOMB ANYWAY?
Evidence Supporting a Nonsterile Intrauterine Environment

In the past it was thought that the fetus and intrauterine environment is sterile, with the newborn's first contact with microbiota occurring at the time of parturition. However, observations arising from healthy pregnancies and studies within relevant animal models have indicated that the fetus may be first exposed to bacteria during gestation.[7,11,22,30–38] Recent studies of the reproductive tract in reproductive-age women show a continuum of microbiota from the vagina, cervix, endometrial lining, and fallopian tubes, indicating a nonsterile intrauterine environment before and during the time of conception, implantation, and placental development.[22,32,33] Other studies using culture-based and polymerase chain reaction (PCR)–based techniques have positively identified bacteria in the fetal membranes, cord blood, and possibly amniotic fluid of healthy, term pregnancies, suggesting that microbiota can inhabit the in utero environment without overtly affecting the pregnancy or the health of the infant.[6–29,34,35,39] In addition, the use of metagenomics sequencing technologies revealed the diversity of the low-biomass microbial community of the placenta parenchyma and chorionic villus,[6] which was also historically considered a sterile tissue in the absence of disease. Across the 320 placentae examined in this study, the most common bacterial taxa were Proteobacteria, such as Escherichia coli, and other microbiota common to the oral cavity, such as Fusobacterium and Streptococcus species.[6] This work has since galvanized efforts to reconsider the fundamental assumptions about when and whence humans first being to acquire microbes in early life. Observations of mother-neonatal pairs by Dong and colleagues[40] and Collado and colleagues[11] showed that the microbiota found within the placenta share significant similarity to that of the neonate's meconium, indicating that microbiota may be additionally transferred across the placenta at the maternal-fetal interface into the fetus, where it would thereafter be presumptively excreted into the amniotic fluid as fetal urine. Of note, in midgestation (17–20 weeks' human gestation), amniotic fluid transitions from being a placental-derived fluid to being composed of fetal urine.

In sum, recent evidence in multiple mammalian systems shows that the female reproductive tract tissues (including the upper vagina and cervix, the uterus, and its endometrial decidua) and placenta are not sterile (**Fig. 1**). Thus, by definition, the womb (uterus) is not sterile. When an embryo of 8 to 16 cells implants in the uterine decidua, and the trophoblasts comprising one-fourth or more of this cell mass begin their process of differentiation and proliferation, they become intimate with the uterine decidua. The subsequent invasion of the spiral arteries facilitates the basis of the

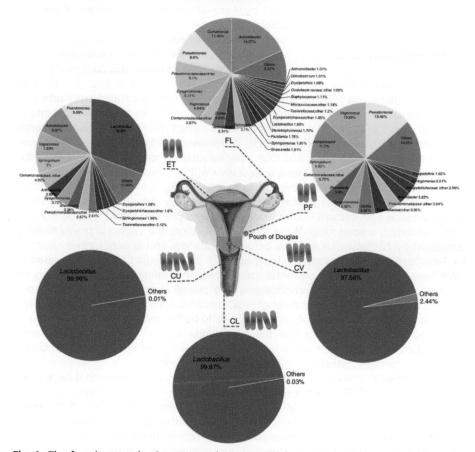

Fig. 1. The female reproductive tract and its associated microbiota. Distinct microbial communities reside in specific sites within the vagina and uterus during pregnancy. These findings indicate a nonsterile environment long before pregnancy and implantation, and thus argue against the sterile-womb theory. For the womb to be sterile during pregnancy, the intimately connected placental villi, parenchyma, and the amnion and chorion would need to exert antimicrobial properties ridding the decidua and tract tissues of their resident communities. It is worth considering the evident constituent and functional overlap between those metagenomes observed in the female reproductive tract and the placenta, chorion-amnion, and amniotic fluid. Emerging themes include what is present, their sparseness and low biomass, as well as their functional capacity. CL, Lower Third of Vagina; CU, Posterior Fornix; CV, Cervical Canal; ET, Endometrium; FL, Fallopian Tube; PF, Peritonial Fluid. (*From* Chen C, Song X, Wei W, et al. The microbiota continuum along the female reproductive tract and its relation to uterine-related diseases. Nature communications. Oct 17 2017;8(1):875; with permission.)

vascular fetal-maternal tissue connection, and is an inherent part of establishing the placenta as more of a conduit than a barrier.[22,41,42]

Supporting evidence has also arisen from multiple animal models. In an early study, Jimenez and colleagues[43] orally administered genetically labeled *Enterococcus faecium* to pregnant mice and sterilely delivered their pups 1 day ahead of anticipated delivery. Interestingly, they could culture and identify the labeled bacterium from the fetal intestine, indicating that microbiota can be transferred from mother to offspring even before delivery occurs.[37] However, the precise route of transmission was not examined and to date remains unclear. Work by Han and colleagues[44] and Fardini and colleagues[45] has put forth a hematogenous model of placental colonization that potentially explains these observations. In the former study, *Fusobacterium nucleatum* was given to pregnant mice intravenously during late gestation (embryonic day 16–17). Although peripheral organs cleared *F nucleatum* within 24 hours, this bacterial species persisted in the placenta and could be detected in the amniotic fluid and fetus at 72 hours postinfection.[45] In the latter study, the investigators intravenously administered commensal bacteria typical of the human oral cavity to pregnant mice late in gestation, and found that they could selectively detect many of these administered microbiota in the placental tissues by PCR.[45] However, the fetal tissues were not specifically examined in this study and thus a hematogenous route of placental and subsequently fetal colonization remains speculative without more definitive evidence.

Ascending colonization from the vagina has been alternatively hypothesized as a potential origin of intrauterine microbes, largely because of its anatomic proximity to the intrauterine environment and its association with preterm birth.[46,47] However, as aforementioned, among most of the human population, the vagina is predominately populated by *Lactobacillus* species before pregnancy, and is only further enriched for lactobacilli as the pregnancy progresses.[48–50] Although *Lactobacillus* species have been detected in the placental membranes in healthy, term pregnancies by metagenomics sequencing methodologies, the overall diversity of commensal species found within the placental parenchyma, amniotic fluid, and neonatal meconium suggests that the vaginal microbiome is unlikely to be the only origin for the full gamut of microbial species found within the intrauterine space.[6–29] Nevertheless, well-designed animal studies are required to further refine these observations and better define a model of microbial transmission during this period.

It is important to consider a limited number of reports and reviews that have challenged the notion that detected metagenomes represent anything beyond environmental or community contamination.[51–56] It is, and remains, the view of our team that the evidence to date is inconclusive as to whether the low-abundance, low-biomass microbiome detected metagenomically represents a live or actively colonizing community. However, given the weighted evidence from dozens of laboratories using multiple and varied techniques, including metagenomics and targeted PCR sequencing, cultivation, microscopy, and cross-validation with human and animal models warrants ongoing consideration and experimental testing because the studies suggesting that detected taxa cannot be distinguished from contaminant controls have several inherent limitations. It is outside the intent and scope of this article to further detail these limitations.

In summary, although the womb has traditionally been considered sterile, this notion is no longer uniformly accepted. Bacteria or their metagenomes have been found in not only the reproductive tissues before pregnancy but the intrauterine tissues of pregnancy.[6–29,57,58] When combined with several recent studies showing the maturation of the fetal gut immune repertoire in this same midgestational interval, it is highly probable that the development of the human microbiome first begins in utero.[59–66] Further evidence for this probability arises from data suggesting that maternal exposures have a lasting impact on the offspring microbiome; this is discussed next.

IS THERE EVIDENCE FOR A ROLE OF MATERNAL EXPOSURES ON THE OFFSPRING'S MICROBIOME?

Impact of Maternal Nutrition in Pregnancy on Offspring Gut Microbiota

The authors have published extensively our findings arising from our nonhuman primate model of maternal high-fat diet feeding, showing that offspring exposed to a high-fat diet in pregnancy show increased anxietylike behaviors, reduced thyroid hormone production, hepatic circadian gene expression, and nonalcoholic fatty liver disease.[67-71] Changes to the fetal epigenome is a likely driver of these observed phenotypes, because there are extensively documented changes to histone acetylation and promotor occupancy around key genes, as well as altered expression of the deacetylase Sirtuin 1 (SIRT1).[67,71-75]

However, diet is also known to be a potent modifier of the gut microbiome, favoring microbiota capable of metabolizing the available substrates.[76] Maternal diet was recently shown to have a long-term impact on the offspring gut microbiome, which may independently contribute to the phenotypes seen or help induce the epigenetic changes previously documented.[77] Dams were either provided a high-fat diet or a control diet before and during pregnancy and lactation. As with humans, a high-fat diet caused significant weight gain and induced corresponding shifts in the nonpregnant gut microbiome.[76,77] To isolate the effects of maternal diet, the offspring of both high-fat and control dams were weaned onto a control diet at 6 to 7 months of age. At 1-year of age, the offspring gut microbiota could be discriminated based on whether their mothers consumed a high-fat or control diet, despite the offspring consuming a control diet for several months.[77] Specifically, a high-fat diet seemed to persistently diminish the relative abundance of commensal *Campylobacter* species in the offspring gut, indicating that maternal diet may play a significant role in shaping the transmission of commensal microbiota that can persist beyond infancy and may extend into adulthood.[77]

The effect of maternal diet seems to extend beyond gestation. Research has shown that a high-fat diet leads to increased milk fat concentration and content compared with a high-carbohydrate diet.[78,79] However, no differences in milk production or quantity of milk were observed. Therefore, neonates consuming breast milk from mothers with a high-fat diet consume a higher energy intake, which can have effects on the development of their microbiome. Although it has not been studied, differences in the properties of the breast milk likely affect which bacteria flourish in the neonatal microbiome, but further studies are needed to confirm this hypothesis. Along these same lines, the maternal diet may be associated with alterations in the breast milk microbiome. However, there currently are no studies published evaluating this association. Investigations in our laboratory are currently exploring this hypothesis and will help us understand any substantial impact the maternal diet has on the breast milk microbiome.

Limited evidence to date has similarly indicated that maternal gestational diet may influence offspring adiposity in early life by altering offspring gut microbiota. Independent studies have implicated certain bacterial species, including *E coli*, as a major modifying factor of this phenotype in the mouse,[80] although it is uncertain whether *E coli* has a similar impact on infant adiposity and growth trajectories in humans or primates. Intriguingly, mitigating the effects of a high-fat diet on the maternal gut microbiota with a prebiotic supplement has been reported to attenuate the impact of maternal diet on the offspring's propensity for adiposity,[30] although our recent work in a nonhuman primate model of a maternal high-fat diet has shown that probiotics do not alter gut microbiome structure, nor do they persist in the gut microbiome.[31] Nevertheless, the development of obesity is an extremely complex pathophysiologic process that may be first programmed in fetal life, but is likely sustained in postnatal life by continued environmental exposure to high-density dietary intake or aberrant microbiota.

In addition to obesity and immunity, recent data suggest that maternal diet may have an impact on offspring behavior by modulating gut microbiota. Bidirectional communication between the brain and the enteric nervous system has long been recognized, but only within the last few years has the impact of gut microbiota been explored in greater detail.[81] By producing neurotransmitters in the gut, such as serotonin or gamma-aminobutyric acid, gut microbiota are hypothesized to contribute to several neurologic and behavioral disorders, including anxiety, depression, and autism, by activating or depressing neural pathways in the enteric and central nervous system.[81] Recent work in the mouse by Buffington and colleagues[82] has indicated that maternal gestational diet may modify offspring behavior by altering offspring gut microbiota in early life. Offspring whose mothers consumed a high-fat diet in pregnancy showed profound social deficits associated with significant changes to oxytocin levels in the brain and specific alterations of the offspring gut microbiota.[82] Intriguingly, postnatal reintroduction of *Lactobacillus reuteri*, which was depleted as a result of a maternal high-fat diet, to the affected offspring was found to ameliorate the deficient social behavior and enhance oxytocin levels in the brain, indicating a causal linkage between maternal diet, gut microbiota, and neurologic development.[82] Thus, future studies examining the impact of maternal gestational diet on offspring gut microbiota will likely continue to refine the understanding of which microbiota are important to neurologic development, how these microbiota are capable of modulating the gut-brain axis, and when these interactions are required.

Preterm Birth

Being born preterm, and the underlying factors leading to a preterm birth, have lasting effects on the short-term and long-term outcomes of neonates.[83] Preterm neonates are at higher risk for infection and intestinal problems, among other illnesses, owing to the lack of sufficient development of host tissues and immaturity of immune regulation at birth. The neonatal microbiome differs in preterm compared with term infants, and it has been hypothesized that some of the disease morbidity association with prematurity is caused by, or exacerbated by, changes in the neonatal microbiome that result from the gestational age at delivery, the underlying predisposing factors, and/or extensive postnatal environmental exposures necessary for preterm neonatal care.[43,84]

Compared with term infants, the gut microbiome of preterm infants tends to be much more sparsely populated. One group of investigators from Spain evaluated 21 premature neonates' intestinal microbiota during the first 3 months of life and compared it with term, exclusively breast-fed, vaginally delivered neonates. Preterm neonates had increased levels of facultative anaerobic microorganisms and decreased levels of strict anaerobes such as *Bifidobacterium*, *Bacteroides*, and *Atopobium*.[85] However, it is difficult to assess whether the changes they found were caused by lack of exclusive human milk feeding (all preterm infants included in this study received mixed feeding) or other associations with hospitalization and/or premature birth itself, such as antibiotics, Furthering the idea that the microbiome is different among premature neonates compared with term neonates, other investigators have shown that very low birth weight neonates (birth weights <1500 g) have decreased diversity of their microbiota, which may be caused by living in a neonatal intensive care unit (NICU), alongside generally continuous antibiotic therapy, sterile isolators, and receipt of parenteral feeds.[86–90]

Not only do premature neonates have a delay in the colonization of "healthy" commensal bacteria, such as *Bifidobacterium*, the premature neonate's microbiota contains higher quantities of pathogenic bacteria. *Klebsiella*, *Weissella*, *Clostridium*, Enterobacteriaceae, Enterococcaceae, Streptococcaceae, and Staphylococcaceae have all been found more commonly in premature neonates' microbiota than in neonates born at term.[32] Concurrent with these results, other investigators found increased levels of *Klebsiella pneumoniae* in the preterm infant microbiota, and *Clostridium difficile* was detected exclusively in the preterm infants.[84,91] These observations may be a result of the types of bacteria that tend to exist in the immediate environment, as well as the sparse microbiome that allows opportunistic colonization. Premature neonates are typically treated in NICUs, which have been shown to harbor a wide range of bacteria, many of which are known opportunistic pathogens that contain antibiotic resistance genes.[92] Many of the neonatal gut microbes can be traced to bacteria found on NICU surfaces, indicating that the environment, in this case, plays a large role in seeding the preterm gut microbiome. Despite this, long-term observations of the preterm gut microbiome have shown that, by 1 to 3 years of age, the preterm microbiome develops similar complexity to term infants, indicating the resilient potential of the gut microbiome.[92] Nevertheless, considering that early life interactions between the host and its microbes are likely critical for crucial patterning, this has the potential to drastically affect a child's long-term health.

In sum, premature neonates are more prone to foster and harbor pathogenic bacteria rather than beneficial commensals, and the diversity and richness of their microbial communities first seen at birth simplifies days to weeks later and following periods of often intense interventions and isolation, as well as antimicrobial therapy. Harboring pathogenic bacteria with less commensal, protective bacteria may be a key reason why this age group has a higher likelihood of necrotizing enterocolitis and other infectious maladies than term neonates.

Human Breast Milk and Formula Feeding

Human milk is a highly complex nutrient source that has multiple nutritive and bioactive components with potential to affect the developing offspring microbiome. Once thought to be sterile, it is now well established that human milk contains a distinct microbiome consisting of diverse species.[93,94] These bacteria seed the gastrointestinal tracts of breastfeeding infants, likely contributing to the significant shifts in microbiome composition associated with breastfeeding. Intriguingly, in addition to skin-associated (*Staphylococcus*) and oral-associated (*Streptococcus*) taxa, the breast milk microbiome includes anaerobic bacteria most commonly associated with the gut, such as *Bifidobacterium* and *Enterococcus*.[93] The origin of these bacteria has yet to be fully elucidated, but evidence suggests that these bacteria may be translocated from the maternal gut via enteromammary trafficking, a pathway in which bacteria in the gut lumen are engulfed by leukocytes through the process of antigen sampling and translocated intracellularly to the mammary glands via systemic circulation.[95]

In support of this hypothesized pathway, a study of mothers given oral *Lactobacillus* probiotics for the treatment of mastitis showed that the *Lactobacillus* strains were detected in the breast milk of 6 out of 10 mothers after oral probiotic administration.[96] Studies of mother-infant pairs have shown that multiple species of bacteria, including gut-associated anaerobes, are common among maternal stool, breast milk, and infant stool, and that the number of shared species between maternal and infant stool significantly increases with time.[97,98] Because profiling by sequencing does not necessarily indicate that transferred bacteria are viable, one study showed that a viable strain of *Bifidobacterium breve* was shared among maternal stool, breast milk, and infant stool from a mother-infant pair.[97] Whatever their origin may be, it is tempting to speculate that these gut-associated bacteria play a key role in establishing the gut microbiome of breastfeeding infants. In addition, because diet is a strong driver of the adult gut microbiome,[76] enteromammary trafficking may represent a mechanism by which dietary-mediated shifts in enteric bacteria are transferred from mother to infant postnatally. However, the effect of maternal diet on the milk microbiome has not been explored and represents a vitally important focus of future research efforts.

Human milk contains many other components with the potential to transmit maternal dietary influence to the offspring microbiome, including macronutrients, human milk oligosaccharides (HMOs), and immune factors such as maternal immunoglobulins (ie, immunoglobulin A [IgA]). High-fat maternal diet significantly affects fat and energy content in human milk, which may in turn affect proliferation of bacteria in the infant gut.[78,99] Human milk contains a high abundance of undigestible oligosaccharides (HMOs) that favor proliferation of specific bacteria in the infant gut, such as *Bifidobacterium* spp.[100] The HMO profile of breast milk varies substantially among women, but the effect of maternal diet on HMO composition has not been well characterized.[100] In addition, human milk contains IgA, which protects nursing infants from infections by providing passive immunity.

Although it is presumed that IgA preferentially targets pathogens, its role in molding the infant gut microbiome has not been well explored. Intriguingly, diet has been shown to modulate IgA production in intestinal and extraintestinal mucosal tissues as well as to alter IgA coating of bacteria in the gut microbiome.[101] Further studies are needed to characterize how diet affects maternal IgA content in human milk and the role of maternal IgA in shaping the offspring gut microbiome.

Mode of Delivery

Women can deliver in one of 2 ways: vaginally or via cesarean delivery. Although one is the often considered the more traditional path and the other is surgical, there is a concern that a lack of exposure to the vaginal microbiome may lead to higher rates of certain diseases occurring later in life, such as atopic conditions, inflammatory bowel disease, type I and II diabetes mellitus, and asthma.[102–105] Given such challenges in establishing a causal relationship between cesarean and later disease, one option is to provide a mechanistic link between the exposure (cesarean) and the outcome (eg, later-life atopic disease). Attempts to do so have led researchers to postulate that absence of vaginal microbes in cases of neonates born via cesarean delivery may be the cause, but how well warranted is this concern?

If the postulate that cesarean-born infants fail to be colonized in their gut (or skin or mouth) by vaginally derived microbes is true, then microbes living in the maternal vaginal niche should (as a rule) establish stable, long-term communities in the infant. However, several lines of evidence have shown this not to be true. First, one of the key tenets of the Human Microbiome Project was the observation of unique body niche speciation. In the vagina, the ecology is dominated by *Lactobacillus* spp, which are highly adept at living at low pH; these same microbes do not dominate the neonatal gut or other body niches. Second, experimental manipulations have not yet provided strong evidence suggesting that vaginal microbes establish long-term community dominance outside the vagina[106] The reasons to perform a cesarean delivery are often clear and evident medical conditions. For instance, conditions such as placenta previa (in which the placenta overlies the cervix) and vasa previa (in which vessels overlie the cervix) are absolute indications for performing cesarean deliveries because, if a vaginal birth occurred, the fetus would likely exsanguinate from severe blood loss. Cesarean delivery would also be performed in women who have a viable fetus and are found to have significant fetal distress necessitating emergent delivery or otherwise face fetal demise. Thus, the reasons for performing cesarean delivery are significantly different compared with allowing the traditional vaginal delivery to occur.

Does a lack of exposure to the vaginal microbiome confer risks to neonates as they grow and develop into adulthood? Some studies have found an association between delivery via cesarean and increased rates of atopic disorders, food allergies, metabolic syndrome, and obesity later in life.[102–105] For instance, a recent large perspective study conducted over 16 years with more than 22,000 participants found that cesarean-delivered infants had a 13% increased risk of obesity later in life.[102] However, how much of that risk can be attributed to the cesarean procedure itself (rather than what led to the cesarean: the maternal indication for cesarean delivery) remains unclear. Investigators studying the human microbiome have attributed these observations to a lack of exposure to the mother's vaginal microbiota(or conversely overt exposure to skin microbiota) during delivery. However, is this assertion confirmed by sound evidence?

Many often-cited studies have not fully elucidated whether it is the mode of delivery versus the underlying indication for delivery that is the culprit. Not all confounders have been thoroughly investigated. For example, in a study by Dominguez-Bello and colleagues,[4] the neonatal microbiome was found to be altered in neonates born via cesarean delivery compared with vaginal delivery. This landmark study created the foundation that the lack of exposure to the maternal vaginal microbiome during parturition (a lack of vaginal seeding) is the cause for these differences.[4] Note that their analysis is based on samples within 5 minutes of delivery and the baby's first stool collected within 24 hours, and thus showcases differences in microbial transmission from the mother to the neonate but does not necessarily reflect true colonization. There are several additional aspects to this particular observational study worth mentioning. First, the study enrolled 9 women and their 10 neonates. Four women and their 4 infants make up the vaginal cohort, whereas 5 women and 6 neonates (1 set of twins) represent the cesarean cohort. Except for the twins, the exact weight of each neonate was not provided, but the methods section of the article states that "[a]ll mothers had healthy pregnancies and all babies were born at term, without complications. Babies weighed between 2 and 5.2 kg (the smallest baby was the twin in second order of birth, after his 3-kg brother)."[4] However, these findings suggest that at least 2 of the pregnancies, likely both cesarean deliveries, were not healthy and uncomplicated." The twins showed significant growth disparity, with a 33% difference in birth weights (2.0 kg vs 3.0 kg). In twins, a discordance of more than 20% is associated with adverse perinatal and postnatal outcomes, and, thus, this is not a healthy and uncomplicated pregnancy. Another neonate in the cohort also had macrosomia, a birth weight of more than 4 kg, which often is found in women who are diabetic. Additional causes include genetic and epigenetic overgrowth disorders, chronic caloric excess, and maternal obesity. Thus, although this study is often cited as showcasing the differences in neonates born via cesarean delivery and those born vaginally, there are at least 3 neonates out of 10 that show signs that the mothers and/or neonates had medical conditions affecting pregnancy.

Our team published one of the first large, prospectively followed cohort of women that includes the maternal indications for delivery along with mode of delivery in evaluating the effects of the development of the neonatal microbiome across multiple body sites.[106] Although neonates born via cesarean delivery have distinct microbiome profiles in the first week of life, this effect did not last past 2 months of age.[106,107] The neonatal microbiome differentiates at specific body sites by 6 to 8 weeks postnatally.[106] Immediately after birth, the mode of delivery was associated with differences in the neonatal microbiome within the nares, skin, and oral cavity. However, the neonatal meconium microbiome clustered separately among cesarean-born infants, suggesting a distinct maternal origin that separated it from the other body sites studied. By 6 weeks of age, the infant microbiota had diversified with body site specificity, and, most remarkably, no differences were identified between infants born via vaginal delivery and those born via cesarean in any of the body sites examined. When these were further parsed by indication for cesarean, or by labored versus unlabored, cesarean-born neonates without labor were the most dissimilar. In addition, when controlling for the indication for delivery and other clinical factors, only maternal diet and formula feeding seem to have a lasting effect on the neonatal microbiome at 6 weeks of age, and the maternal indication for delivery plays a significant role in this development. Along these lines, in preterm neonates, other investigators have shown that tracheal aspirates have been evaluated for the evaluation of the microbiome, and there no appreciable differences between those premature neonates born via cesarean delivery versus those born vaginally.[108] The recent The Environmental Determinants of Diabetes in the Young (TEDDY) Study cohort studies further failed to delineate a fundamental role for cesarean delivery in shaping the early developmental microbiome.

In sum, although others have previously observed that neonates born vaginally or vaginally seeded showed increased *Lactobacillus* and *Bacteroides*, Chu and colleagues[106,107] found low levels of *Bacteroides* and/or high levels of *Lactobacillus* to be equally probable in vaginally and cesarean-delivered neonates and infants, but their variation depended on several other collinear factors, such as the percentage of fat in the maternal diet, formula feeding, labored versus unlabored delivery, and gestational age at delivery. These observations were consistent with much earlier studies showing that vaginal delivery rarely transfers *Lactobacillus* to the neonate, and have hence been recapitulated by multiple groups that collectively failed to show a significant or lasting distinction in the gut microbiota of vaginal-delivered versus cesarean-delivered infants or children. Based on the emerging data in well-designed, prospective, and population-based cohorts, the authors conclude that it is highly probable that the maternal indication for cesarean delivery plays a larger role than the mode of delivery itself. This possibility renders the alternate view that a lack of vaginal seeding[109,110] by the maternal vaginal microbiome during parturition is unlikely to be the key the culprit in any subsequent association between cesarean birth and disease later in life. The origin of the risk lies in the maternal "soil" from which the neonate originated (ie, the maternal and intrauterine milieu). Although these may or may not be the indications that led to the decision to perform a cesarean delivery, parsing cause from surgery is of fundamental importance because the nature and timing of any corrective interventions are widely different.

FUTURE DIRECTIONS AND SUMMARY
Future Directions

Future studies expanding on the work presented in this article should focus on 3 major directions: (1) determining the impact of a maternal high-fat diet–associated gut microbiome on the immune and behavioral phenotype of the offspring, (2) identifying the corresponding effect of maternal diet on the offspring gut microbiome during breastfeeding, and (3) further characterizing and identifying the major bacterial and host mediators of maternal-fetal bacterial transmission. Given that any initial differences in the infant microbiota between vaginal and cesarean delivery become less profound over time, it remains unclear how birth mode influences the risk factors for disease by modulation of the microbiota. This question is of paramount importance for mothers to make informed decisions regarding the desired birth mode.

It is similarly crucially important to understand the impact the maternal diet (independent of obesity and weight gain or loss in pregnancy) has on her developing offspring, its microbiome, and its lifelong risk of metabolic disease. Although clinicians cannot merely blame the mothers for any adversity their children experience in life, they can and must provide sound evidence on those factors that the mothers can control and modify during their pregnancies. Pregnant woman cannot safely lose dozens of kilograms of weight necessary to transition from being obese to normal weight in the span of 10, 20, or even 40 weeks. However, they can make conscious decision regarding the quality of their diets. More importantly, given the association between social disparities, diet, and health outcomes, clinicians can make informed public health decisions regarding the importance of providing high-quality and nutritional food during pregnancy.

As one such example, the authors have previously established within our nonhuman primate model that a maternal high-fat gestational diet (but not maternal obesity per se) results in changes to the metabolic profile and epigenome of the offspring.[67,70,71] Ongoing work within this model has focused on characterizing additional phenotypes within these animals likely mediated by an altered gut microbiome. This work includes prior and continuing studies that have documented abnormal behavioral tendencies within offspring exposed to a maternal high-fat gestational diet.[73,75] Future studies examining key gut bacteria and their metabolites altered by a maternal high-fat diet will be required to understand how gut microbiota can influence behavior by acting on the gut-brain-axis.[81] It is possible that gut microbiota either produce key regulators that alter neuronal transmission or indirectly influence the production of key neuropeptides. Therefore, multiomics using relevant dyad models will be crucially important in the future. Along these lines, prior evidence has indicated that microbes are essential for patterning methylation and histone modifications of key components of innate and adaptive immunity, including TLR4 and Th17 balance.[111–114] Studying host responses to the presence or absence of differentially associated bacteria within this ex vivo condition may reveal key host-microbial interactions essential for proper immune development within the gut.

Additional studies are required to determine the relative impact of maternal diet during breastfeeding, and to tease apart the intrauterine exposure risks from the early ex utero risks. It is challenging, if not impossible, to cross-foster primate offspring because of high-rates of infanticide, and generally unacceptable in human clinical studies. As a result, it is not possible to distinguish between the gestational and lactational periods. Breast milk harbors a unique microbiome that changes through time postnatally. Notably, the composition of breast milk has been shown to change with maternal diet,[78] and ongoing work within our laboratory has shown additional changes in the microbiome composition. It is therefore possible that maternal diet in lactation has an additional or synergistic effect on the offspring gut microbiome. Innovative paired study designs in human trials may be beneficial in parsing out the relative impacts of gestational versus lactational exposures over time.

SUMMARY

Although parturition was traditionally assumed to be the first point at which neonates are exposed to microbes, emerging evidence indicates that this is unlikely to be true.

The presence of microbes and low-biomass microbial communities within the intra-uterine space (the uterine decidua, the placenta and the amnion and chorionic membranes, and amniotic fluid) has now been consistently documented in a growing multitude of mammalian species. Right at birth, distinct microbial communities in the meconium among preterm and healthy-term neonates have been detected and described, and these impressively expand in the first days to weeks of life to readily show discrete body niche communities long before that same infant alters its diet or engages in meaningful contact with the outside world (**Fig. 2**). In addition, although it has been appreciated for more than a century that congenital viruses are vertically

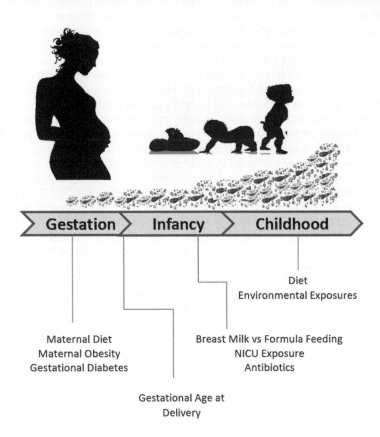

Factors Affecting Development of the Human Microbiome

Fig. 2. Factors reported to affect the acquisition and development of the gut microbiome. Numerous reports have observed an effect of both internal characteristics and external factors on the characteristics of the neonatal, infant, and early childhood microbiome. Adulthood and infancy, which encompasses the first year of life, have been the 2 predominately studied time periods. More recent reports have shown an effect of gestational exposures, including maternal obesity status and gestational diabetes. In the future, fundamentally crucial developmental windows to study will include the period of acquiring reproductive competence (periadolescence, adolescence, and early reproductive age) as well as the intervals immediately before and including pregnancy.

transmitted from mother to fetus, it remains a consistent observation from human immunodeficiency virus to Zika that only a small fraction become infected in utero. In recent months, it has been suggested that bacteria may play a role in regulating intrauterine viral transmission, although the mechanisms by which this might occur are presently unknown.

Although some key questions have been answered regarding the development of the human microbiome and its impact on human disease, much still remains unknown. Physicians and scientist alike must seek answers to these vital questions in order to elucidate potential causes for disease states, including those that arise because of aberrant development of the human microbiome and thus can be amenable to therapies early in life. Moreover, continuing to operate under age-old paradigms of "purity at birth," which ignore mounting evidence for low-biomass metagenomes (be they of sparse abundance or not) in favor of a priori assumptions, will limit progress. Although our laboratory presently remains agnostic as to the issue of whether these consistently observed low-biomass communities are alive and colonize the fetus, or alternately enable later colonization through a process of immune tolerance, we look forward to future and bold science that will help elucidate one of the most significant questions of our time. In the interval until that occurs, clinicians must remain both open-minded and constructively critical of the available evidence.

ACKNOWLEDGMENTS

We would like to acknowledge our funding is through the National Institutes of Health through the following two grants: 6R01 DK089201 and 1R01 HD091731.

REFERENCES

1. Sender R, Fuchs S, Milo R. Revised estimates for the number of human and bacteria cells in the body. PLoS Biol 2016;14(8):e1002533.
2. Human Microbiome Project Consortium. Structure, function and diversity of the healthy human microbiome. Nature 2012;486(7402):207–14.
3. Biasucci G, Rubini M, Riboni S, et al. Mode of delivery affects the bacterial community in the newborn gut. Early Hum Dev 2010;86(Suppl 1):13–5.
4. Dominguez-Bello MG, Costello EK, Contreras M, et al. Delivery mode shapes the acquisition and structure of the initial microbiota across multiple body habitats in newborns. Proc Natl Acad Sci U S A 2010;107(26):11971–5.
5. Zhu L, Luo F, Hu W, et al. Bacterial communities in the womb during healthy pregnancy. Front Microbiol 2018;9:2163.
6. Aagaard K, Ma J, Antony KM, et al. The placenta harbors a unique microbiome. Sci Transl Med 2014;6(237):237ra265.
7. Doyle RM, Alber DG, Jones HE, et al. Term and preterm labour are associated with distinct microbial community structures in placental membranes which are independent of mode of delivery. Placenta 2014;35(12):1099–101.
8. Antony KM, Ma J, Mitchell KB, et al. The preterm placental microbiome varies in association with excess maternal gestational weight gain. Am J Obstet Gynecol 2015;212(5):653.e1-16.
9. Zheng J, Xiao X, Zhang Q, et al. The placental microbiome varies in association with low birth weight in full-term neonates. Nutrients 2015;7(8):6924–37.
10. Bassols J, Serino M, Carreras-Badosa G, et al. Gestational diabetes is associated with changes in placental microbiota and microbiome. Pediatr Res 2016; 80(6):777–84.

11. Collado MC, Rautava S, Aakko J, et al. Human gut colonisation may be initiated in utero by distinct microbial communities in the placenta and amniotic fluid. Sci Rep 2016;6:23129.

12. Prince AL, Ma J, Kannan PS, et al. The placental membrane microbiome is altered among subjects with spontaneous preterm birth with and without chorioamnionitis. Am J Obstet Gynecol 2016;214(5):627.e1-e16.

13. Doyle RM, Harris K, Kamiza S, et al. Bacterial communities found in placental tissues are associated with severe chorioamnionitis and adverse birth outcomes. PLoS One 2017;12(7):e0180167.

14. Parnell LA, Briggs CM, Cao B, et al. Microbial communities in placentas from term normal pregnancy exhibit spatially variable profiles. Sci Rep 2017;7(1): 11200.

15. Gomez-Arango LF, Barrett HL, McIntyre HD, et al. Contributions of the maternal oral and gut microbiome to placental microbial colonization in overweight and obese pregnant women. Sci Rep 2017;7(1):2860.

16. Zheng J, Xiao XH, Zhang Q, et al. Correlation of placental microbiota with fetal macrosomia and clinical characteristics in mothers and newborns. Oncotarget 2017;8(47):82314-25.

17. Leon LJ, Doyle R, Diez-Benavente E, et al. Enrichment of clinically relevant organisms in spontaneous preterm delivered placenta and reagent contamination across all clinical groups in a large UK pregnancy cohort. Appl Environ Microbiol 2018;84(14) [pii:e00483-18].

18. Mitchell CM, Haick A, Nkwopara E, et al. Colonization of the upper genital tract by vaginal bacterial species in nonpregnant women. Am J Obstet Gynecol 2015;212(5):611.e1-9.

19. Franasiak JM, Werner MD, Juneau CR, et al. Endometrial microbiome at the time of embryo transfer: next-generation sequencing of the 16S ribosomal subunit. J Assist Reprod Genet 2016;33(1):129-36.

20. Moreno I, Codoner FM, Vilella F, et al. Evidence that the endometrial microbiota has an effect on implantation success or failure. Am J Obstet Gynecol 2016; 215(6):684-703.

21. Verstraelen H, Vilchez-Vargas R, Desimpel F, et al. Characterisation of the human uterine microbiome in non-pregnant women through deep sequencing of the V1-2 region of the 16S rRNA gene. PeerJ 2016;4:e1602.

22. Chen C, Song X, Wei W, et al. The microbiota continuum along the female reproductive tract and its relation to uterine-related diseases. Nat Commun 2017; 8(1):875.

23. Kyono K, Hashimoto T, Nagai Y, et al. Analysis of endometrial microbiota by 16S ribosomal RNA gene sequencing among infertile patients: a single-center pilot study. Reprod Med Biol 2018;17(3):297-306.

24. Prince AL, Chu DM, Seferovic MD, et al. The perinatal microbiome and pregnancy: moving beyond the vaginal microbiome. Cold Spring Harb Perspect Med 2015;5(6) [pii:a023051].

25. Prince AL, Antony KM, Ma J, et al. The microbiome and development: a mother's perspective. Semin Reprod Med 2014;32(1):14-22.

26. Giudice LC. Challenging dogma: the endometrium has a microbiome with functional consequences! Am J Obstet Gynecol 2016;215(6):682-3.

27. Moreno I, Franasiak JM. Endometrial microbiota-new player in town. Fertil Steril 2017;108(1):32-9.

28. Pelzer E, Gomez-Arango LF, Barrett HL, et al. Review: maternal health and the placental microbiome. Placenta 2017;54:30-7.

29. Benner M, Ferwerda G, Joosten I, et al. How uterine microbiota might be responsible for a receptive, fertile endometrium. Hum Reprod Update 2018; 24(4):393–415.
30. Paul HA, Bomhof MR, Vogel HJ, et al. Diet-induced changes in maternal gut microbiota and metabolomic profiles influence programming of offspring obesity risk in rats. Sci Rep 2016;6:20683.
31. Pace RM, Prince AL, Ma J, et al. Modulations in the offspring gut microbiome are refractory to postnatal synbiotic supplementation among juvenile primates. BMC Microbiol 2018;18(1):28.
32. Baker JM, Chase DM, Herbst-Kralovetz MM. Uterine microbiota: residents, tourists, or invaders? Front Immunol 2018;9:208.
33. Seo SS, Arokiyaraj S, Kim MK, et al. High prevalence of leptotrichia amnionii, atopobium vaginae, sneathia sanguinegens, and factor 1 microbes and association of spontaneous abortion among Korean women. Biomed Res Int 2017; 2017:5435089.
34. Dong Y, St Clair PJ, Ramzy I, et al. A microbiologic and clinical study of placental inflammation at term. Obstet Gynecol 1987;70(2):175–82.
35. Cao B, Mysorekar IU. Intracellular bacteria in placental basal plate localize to extravillous trophoblasts. Placenta 2014;35(2):139–42.
36. Perez-Munoz ME, Arrieta MC, Ramer-Tait AE, et al. A critical assessment of the "sterile womb" and "in utero colonization" hypotheses: implications for research on the pioneer infant microbiome. Microbiome 2017;5(1):48.
37. Jimenez E, Marin ML, Martin R, et al. Is meconium from healthy newborns actually sterile? Res Microbiol 2008;159(3):187–93.
38. Blaser MJ, Dominguez-Bello MG. The human microbiome before birth. Cell Host Microbe 2016;20(5):558–60.
39. Mysorekar IU, Cao B. Microbiome in parturition and preterm birth. Semin Reprod Med 2014;32(1):50–5.
40. Dong XD, Li XR, Luan JJ, et al. Bacterial communities in neonatal feces are similar to mothers' placentae. Can J Infect Dis Med Microbiol 2015;26(2):90–4.
41. Ding T, Schloss PD. Dynamics and associations of microbial community types across the human body. Nature 2014;509(7500):357–60.
42. Pelzer ES, Allan JA, Waterhouse MA, et al. Microorganisms within human follicular fluid: effects on IVF. PLoS One 2013;8(3):e59062.
43. Jimenez E, Fernandez L, Marin ML, et al. Isolation of commensal bacteria from umbilical cord blood of healthy neonates born by Cesarean section. Curr Microbiol 2005;51(4):270–4.
44. Han YW, Redline RW, Li M, et al. Fusobacterium nucleatum induces premature and term stillbirths in pregnant mice: implication of oral bacteria in preterm birth. Infect Immun 2004;72(4):2272–9.
45. Fardini Y, Chung P, Dumm R, et al. Transmission of diverse oral bacteria to murine placenta: evidence for the oral microbiome as a potential source of intrauterine infection. Infect Immun 2010;78(4):1789–96.
46. Usui R, Ohkuchi A, Matsubara S, et al. Vaginal lactobacilli and preterm birth. J Perinat Med 2002;30(6):458–66.
47. Kindinger LM, Bennett PR, Lee YS, et al. The interaction between vaginal microbiota, cervical length, and vaginal progesterone treatment for preterm birth risk. Microbiome 2017;5(1):6.
48. Aagaard K, Riehle K, Ma J, et al. A metagenomic approach to characterization of the vaginal microbiome signature in pregnancy. PLoS One 2012;7(6):e36466.

49. Walther-Antonio MR, Jeraldo P, Berg Miller ME, et al. Pregnancy's stronghold on the vaginal microbiome. PLoS One 2014;9(6):e98514.
50. MacIntyre DA, Chandiramani M, Lee YS, et al. The vaginal microbiome during pregnancy and the postpartum period in a European population. Sci Rep 2015;5:8988.
51. Theis KR, Romero R, Winters AD, et al. Does the human placenta delivered at term have a microbiota? Results of cultivation, quantitative real-time PCR, 16S rRNA gene sequencing, and metagenomics. Am J Obstet Gynecol 2019; 220(3):267.e1-e39.
52. Lauder AP, Roche AM, Sherrill-Mix S, et al. Comparison of placenta samples with contamination controls does not provide evidence for a distinct placenta microbiota. Microbiome 2016;4(1):29.
53. Kim D, Hofstaedter CE, Zhao C, et al. Optimizing methods and dodging pitfalls in microbiome research. Microbiome 2017;5(1):52.
54. Bushman FD. De-discovery of the placenta microbiome. Am J Obstet Gynecol 2019;220(3):213-4.
55. Leiby JS, McCormick K, Sherrill-Mix S, et al. Lack of detection of a human placenta microbiome in samples from preterm and term deliveries. Microbiome 2018;6(1):196.
56. Glassing A, Dowd SE, Galandiuk S, et al. Inherent bacterial DNA contamination of extraction and sequencing reagents may affect interpretation of microbiota in low bacterial biomass samples. Gut Pathog 2016;8:24.
57. Cao B, Stout MJ, Lee I, et al. Placental microbiome and its role in preterm birth. Neoreviews 2014;15(12):e537-45.
58. Stout MJ, Zhou Y, Wylie KM, et al. Early pregnancy vaginal microbiome trends and preterm birth. Am J Obstet Gynecol 2017;217(3):356.e1-e18.
59. Backhed F, Roswall J, Peng Y, et al. Dynamics and stabilization of the human gut microbiome during the first year of life. Cell Host Microbe 2015;17(6):852.
60. Matamoros S, Gras-Leguen C, Le Vacon F, et al. Development of intestinal microbiota in infants and its impact on health. Trends Microbiol 2013;21(4):167-73.
61. Mackie RI, Sghir A, Gaskins HR. Developmental microbial ecology of the neonatal gastrointestinal tract. Am J Clin Nutr 1999;69(5):1035S-45S.
62. Stewart CJ, Ajami NJ, O'Brien JL, et al. Temporal development of the gut microbiome in early childhood from the TEDDY study. Nature 2018;562(7728):583-8.
63. Stewart CJ, Embleton ND, Clements E, et al. Cesarean or vaginal birth does not impact the longitudinal development of the gut microbiome in a cohort of exclusively preterm infants. Front Microbiol 2017;8:1008.
64. Stewart CJ, Embleton ND, Marrs EC, et al. Temporal bacterial and metabolic development of the preterm gut reveals specific signatures in health and disease. Microbiome 2016;4(1):67.
65. Stewart CJ, Embleton ND, Marrs ECL, et al. Longitudinal development of the gut microbiome and metabolome in preterm neonates with late onset sepsis and healthy controls. Microbiome 2017;5(1):75.
66. Vebo HC, Sekelja M, Nestestog R, et al. Temporal development of the infant gut microbiota in immunoglobulin E-sensitized and nonsensitized children determined by the GA-map infant array. Clin Vaccine Immunol 2011;18(8):1326-35.
67. Suter M, Bocock P, Showalter L, et al. Epigenomics: maternal high-fat diet exposure in utero disrupts peripheral circadian gene expression in nonhuman primates. FASEB J 2011;25(2):714-26.
68. Suter MA, Aagaard-Tillery KM. Environmental influences on epigenetic profiles. Semin Reprod Med 2009;27(5):380-90.

69. Suter MA, Chen A, Burdine MS, et al. A maternal high-fat diet modulates fetal SIRT1 histone and protein deacetylase activity in nonhuman primates. FASEB J 2012;26(12):5106–14.
70. Suter MA, Sangi-Haghpeykar H, Showalter L, et al. Maternal high-fat diet modulates the fetal thyroid axis and thyroid gene expression in a nonhuman primate model. Mol Endocrinol 2012;26(12):2071–80.
71. Suter MA, Takahashi D, Grove KL, et al. Postweaning exposure to a high-fat diet is associated with alterations to the hepatic histone code in Japanese macaques. Pediatr Res 2013;74(3):252–8.
72. Suter M, Abramovici A, Aagaard-Tillery K. Genetic and epigenetic influences associated with intrauterine growth restriction due to in utero tobacco exposure. Pediatr Endocrinol Rev 2010;8(2):94–102.
73. Sullivan EL, Grayson B, Takahashi D, et al. Chronic consumption of a high-fat diet during pregnancy causes perturbations in the serotonergic system and increased anxiety-like behavior in nonhuman primate offspring. J Neurosci 2010;30(10):3826–30.
74. Thorn SR, Baquero KC, Newsom SA, et al. Early life exposure to maternal insulin resistance has persistent effects on hepatic NAFLD in juvenile nonhuman primates. Diabetes 2014;63(8):2702–13.
75. Sullivan EL, Smith MS, Grove KL. Perinatal exposure to high-fat diet programs energy balance, metabolism and behavior in adulthood. Neuroendocrinology 2011;93(1):1–8.
76. David LA, Maurice CF, Carmody RN, et al. Diet rapidly and reproducibly alters the human gut microbiome. Nature 2014;505(7484):559–63.
77. Ma J, Prince AL, Bader D, et al. High-fat maternal diet during pregnancy persistently alters the offspring microbiome in a primate model. Nat Commun 2014;5: 3889.
78. Mohammad MA, Sunehag AL, Haymond MW. Effect of dietary macronutrient composition under moderate hypocaloric intake on maternal adaptation during lactation. Am J Clin Nutr 2009;89(6):1821–7.
79. Munch EM, Harris RA, Mohammad M, et al. Transcriptome profiling of microRNA by Next-Gen deep sequencing reveals known and novel miRNA species in the lipid fraction of human breast milk. PLoS One 2013;8(2):e50564.
80. Fak F, Karlsson CL, Ahrne S, et al. Effects of a high-fat diet during pregnancy and lactation are modulated by E. coli in rat offspring. Int J Obes 2012;36(5): 744–51.
81. Foster JA, McVey Neufeld KA. Gut-brain axis: how the microbiome influences anxiety and depression. Trends Neurosci 2013;36(5):305–12.
82. Buffington SA, Di Prisco GV, Auchtung TA, et al. Microbial reconstitution reverses maternal diet-induced social and synaptic deficits in offspring. Cell 2016;165(7):1762–75.
83. Saigal S, Doyle LW. An overview of mortality and sequelae of preterm birth from infancy to adulthood. Lancet 2008;371(9608):261–9.
84. Moles L, Gomez M, Jimenez E, et al. Preterm infant gut colonization in the neonatal ICU and complete restoration 2 years later. Clin Microbiol Infect 2015;21(10):936.e1-10.
85. Arboleya S, Binetti A, Salazar N, et al. Establishment and development of intestinal microbiota in preterm neonates. FEMS Microbiol Ecol 2012;79(3):763–72.
86. Rouge C, Goldenberg O, Ferraris L, et al. Investigation of the intestinal microbiota in preterm infants using different methods. Anaerobe 2010;16(4):362–70.

87. Roudiere L, Jacquot A, Marchandin H, et al. Optimized PCR-temporal temperature gel electrophoresis compared to cultivation to assess diversity of gut microbiota in neonates. J Microbiol Methods 2009;79(2):156–65.

88. Magne F, Abely M, Boyer F, et al. Low species diversity and high interindividual variability in faeces of preterm infants as revealed by sequences of 16S rRNA genes and PCR-temporal temperature gradient gel electrophoresis profiles. FEMS Microbiol Ecol 2006;57(1):128–38.

89. Schwartz S, Friedberg I, Ivanov IV, et al. A metagenomic study of diet-dependent interaction between gut microbiota and host in infants reveals differences in immune response. Genome Biol 2012;13(4):r32.

90. Neu J. Intestinal microbiota studies in preterm infants. J Pediatr Gastroenterol Nutr 2016;62(2):193–4.

91. Gibson MK, Wang B, Ahmadi S, et al. Developmental dynamics of the preterm infant gut microbiota and antibiotic resistome. Nat Microbiol 2016;1:16024.

92. Brooks B, Firek BA, Miller CS, et al. Microbes in the neonatal intensive care unit resemble those found in the gut of premature infants. Microbiome 2014;2(1):1.

93. Hunt KM, Foster JA, Forney LJ, et al. Characterization of the diversity and temporal stability of bacterial communities in human milk. PLoS One 2011;6(6): e21313.

94. Khodayar-Pardo P, Mira-Pascual L, Collado MC, et al. Impact of lactation stage, gestational age and mode of delivery on breast milk microbiota. J Perinatol 2014;34(8):599–605.

95. Latuga MS, Stuebe A, Seed PC. A review of the source and function of microbiota in breast milk. Semin Reprod Med 2014;32(1):68–73.

96. Jimenez E, Fernandez L, Maldonado A, et al. Oral administration of Lactobacillus strains isolated from breast milk as an alternative for the treatment of infectious mastitis during lactation. Appl Environ Microbiol 2008;74(15):4650–5.

97. Jost T, Lacroix C, Braegger CP, et al. Vertical mother-neonate transfer of maternal gut bacteria via breastfeeding. Environ Microbiol 2014;16(9): 2891–904.

98. Schanche M, Avershina E, Dotterud C, et al. High-resolution analyses of overlap in the microbiota between mothers and their children. Curr Microbiol 2015;71(2): 283–90.

99. Robinson DT, Caplan MS. Linking fat intake, the intestinal microbiome, and necrotizing enterocolitis in premature infants. Pediatr Res 2015;77(1–2):121–6.

100. Bode L. Human milk oligosaccharides: every baby needs a sugar mama. Glycobiology 2012;22(9):1147–62.

101. Massot-Cladera M, Abril-Gil M, Torres S, et al. Impact of cocoa polyphenol extracts on the immune system and microbiota in two strains of young rats. Br J Nutr 2014;112(12):1944–54.

102. Yuan C, Gaskins AJ, Blaine AI, et al. Association between cesarean birth and risk of obesity in offspring in childhood, adolescence, and early adulthood. JAMA Pediatr 2016;170(11):e162385.

103. Cardwell CR, Stene LC, Joner G, et al. Caesarean section is associated with an increased risk of childhood-onset type 1 diabetes mellitus: a meta-analysis of observational studies. Diabetologia 2008;51(5):726–35.

104. Kolokotroni O, Middleton N, Gavatha M, et al. Asthma and atopy in children born by caesarean section: effect modification by family history of allergies - a population based cross-sectional study. BMC Pediatr 2012;12:179.

105. Sevelsted A, Stokholm J, Bisgaard H. Risk of asthma from cesarean delivery depends on membrane rupture. J Pediatr 2016;171:38–42.e1-4.

106. Chu DM, Ma J, Prince AL, et al. Maturation of the infant microbiome community structure and function across multiple body sites and in relation to mode of delivery. Nat Med 2017;23(3):314–26.
107. Chu DM, Meyer KM, Prince AL, et al. Impact of maternal nutrition in pregnancy and lactation on offspring gut microbial composition and function. Gut Microbes 2016;7(6):459–70.
108. Lohmann P, Luna RA, Hollister EB, et al. The airway microbiome of intubated premature infants: characteristics and changes that predict the development of bronchopulmonary dysplasia. Pediatr Res 2014;76(3):294–301.
109. Committee on Obstetric Practice. Committee Opinion No. 725: vaginal seeding. Obstet Gynecol 2017;130(5):e274–8.
110. Dominguez-Bello MG, De Jesus-Laboy KM, Shen N, et al. Partial restoration of the microbiota of Cesarean-born infants via vaginal microbial transfer. Nat Med 2016;22(3):250–3.
111. Takahashi K, Sugi Y, Hosono A, et al. Epigenetic regulation of TLR4 gene expression in intestinal epithelial cells for the maintenance of intestinal homeostasis. J Immunol 2009;183(10):6522–9.
112. Tan Y, Zou KF, Qian W, et al. Expression and implication of toll-like receptors TLR2, TLR4 and TLR9 in colonic mucosa of patients with ulcerative colitis. J Huazhong Univ Sci Technolog Med Sci 2014;34(5):785–90.
113. Ivanov II, Atarashi K, Manel N, et al. Induction of intestinal Th17 cells by segmented filamentous bacteria. Cell 2009;139(3):485–98.
114. Gomez de Aguero M, Ganal-Vonarburg SC, Fuhrer T, et al. The maternal microbiota drives early postnatal innate immune development. Science 2016; 351(6279):1296–302.

The Human Microbiota and Its Relationship with Allergies

Nanna Fyhrquist, PhD[a,b],*

KEYWORDS

- Allergic disease • Human microbiota • Dysbiosis • Biodiversity hypothesis

KEY POINTS

- Perturbations in the human microbiome may have profound effects on the host, which may result in developing chronic inflammation and disease, especially in genetically predisposed individuals.
- The mechanisms via which the human microbiota may be regulating the immune system, either by providing protective signals or stimulating effector mechanisms, are only beginning to be understood.
- Many allergic conditions are associated with dysbiosis; however, it remains unclear whether it is the cause or an epiphenomenon of the disease.

INTRODUCTION

Trillions of microorganisms thrive on and inside bodies and have done so, participating in the shaping of physiology through millions of years of common evolution. The relationship between humans and their microbiota is truly mutualistic, with microorganisms playing a significant role in host digestion, metabolism, and the immune system. Several lines of evidence indicate that the human-associated microbes have been selected based on coadaptation.[1] Initially, microorganisms were regarded as mere pathogens, which cause infections and disease and which the host immune system should recognize and eliminate. It has become increasingly clear, however, that microorganisms influence most aspects of human physiology, and, conversely, the host immune system has largely developed to support the mutualistic relationship between the host and these highly diverse microbes. This interaction is extensive, as

Disclosure Statement: Dr. N. Fyhrquist received funding support from Svenska kulturfonden, the Jane and Aatos Erkko Foundation and the FP7/2007-2013 grant 261366.
[a] Institute of Environmental Medicine, Karolinska Institutet, Box 210, Stockholm 17177, Sweden; [b] Department of Bacteriology and Immunology, Medicum, University of Helsinki, Helsinki, Finland
* IMM, Box 210, Stockholm 17177, Sweden.
E-mail address: nanna.fyhrquist@ki.se

evidenced by a study comparing germ-free mice with conventionally raised mice, revealing that most metabolites in host blood are derived from the gut microbiota.[2] Therefore, significant perturbations in the microbial community, or dysbioses, may have profound effects on the host, which may result in developing chronic inflammation and disease, especially in genetically predisposed individuals.

The composition of the human microbiota is largely determined by anatomic site, with some interpersonal variation. Thus, individuals can be grouped according to the occurrence of major phyla at specific body sites. Moreover, there is temporal variability in the composition, influenced by diet, season, or changes in the state of physiology, including regularly occurring fluctuations, such as the menses, or isolated phenomena, such as pregnancy.[3,4] Nevertheless, the microbiota of 1 individual usually varies fairly narrowly, except when significantly perturbed by agents, such as antibiotic treatments or infections. Such episodes can lead to a new transient equilibrium or even a new stable state. The concept of resilience, that is, the capacity of an ecosystem to recover from perturbations, is central in the context of health and the human microbiota. Although adult microbiotas usually are highly resilient, children are more vulnerable, and frequent perturbations may lead to increasingly impaired recovery each time, with implications for health.

Chronic inflammatory diseases are on the rise worldwide today; the central role of the immune system in driving disease is only beginning to be understood. Yet, how the environment, including the human microbiota, may trigger this development, is unknown. For many conditions and illnesses, a challenge is to discover whether there is a causal link between variations in the microbiota and pathology. It has been hypothesized that although human ecology changes, so does the microbiota, with implications for health. A modern lifestyle, including large-scale urban living, cesarean sections, replacement of breast milk with formula, cleaner drinking water, smaller families, and frequent antibiotics, has brought with it dramatic changes to the transmission and maintenance of the indigenous microbiota, resulting in long-term effects on its composition and stability. And if the microbiota affects physiology, and its composition has changed, it should be no surprise that this might alter host homeostasis and, as a consequence, disease risk.[5]

ALLERGIES AND IMMUNOREGULATION BY THE HUMAN RESIDENTIAL MICROBIOTA

Allergic diseases, including asthma, rhinitis, atopic dermatitis (AD), and food allergies, have been increasing to epidemic proportions during the past century, especially in high-income countries. The idea that there might be a link between the allergy epidemic and reduced microbial exposure was first proposed in 1989. The so-called hygiene hypothesis, formulated by Dr David Strachan,[6] suggested that a lower frequency of infections in early childhood could explain the rise in atopic diseases during the twentieth century. Later on, the hygiene hypothesis was refined to include the old friends hypothesis,[7] which suggests that it is not the infections that protect against allergies; rather, the allergy epidemic is a result of a loss of sufficient interaction with health-promoting microbes—old friends—which have been present through thousands of years of common evolution and the evolvement of the mammalian immune system. Moreover, the hygiene hypothesis was expanded in 2010 by von Hertzen and colleagues[8] into the biodiversity hypothesis, which suggests that, in addition to microbes in the home, in food, in drinking water, and on domestic animals, microbes of the living environment, in general, may play a key role in shaping the composition of microbial communities on the skin, in the respiratory system, and in the gut, with consequences for physiology and health.

Old friends include usually nonharmful commensals, with which humans coevolved, because they performed crucial physiologic functions. Moreover, humans evolved to tolerate other harmless organisms, which inevitably were taken daily into the body in large quantities, and also organisms that induced low-level infections but were tolerated, such as helminths, *Salmonella*, hepatitis A virus, and *Helicobacter. pylori*. Some of these organisms, such as blood nematodes, can be harmful, but, once established, trying to eliminate them may cause pointless immunopathology. These microbes continuously stimulate the immune system via microbe-associated molecular patterns or pathogen-associated molecular patterns and cognate pattern recognition receptors, and it is natural to conceive that the immune system evolved to detect and eliminate these potentially dangerous organisms. What is less obvious, however, is that microbial exposures at the same time also serve to down-regulate the immune system, preventing it from developing inappropriate inflammatory responses against self, harmless allergens, and gut contents. These are all targets in autoimmune diseases, allergic disorders, and inflammatory bowel diseases. Moreover, the regulatory mechanisms should be able to shut down ongoing inflammatory responses and down-regulate unnecessary background inflammation.[9]

The mechanisms via which the human residential microbiota may be regulating the immune system are only beginning to be understood. These include secreted molecules or metabolites, such as short-chain fatty acids (SCFAs), which can induce the differentiation of regulatory dendritic cells (DCs) or the expansion of regulatory T-cell (Treg) populations.[10,11] Moreover, microbes can influence the immune system through the induction of helper T cell type 1 (T_H)-type immune responses, which inhibit the development of T_H2 cells and thereby protect against helper T cell type 2 (T_H2)-driven allergies. Endotoxins stimulate macrophages and antigen-presenting cells to produce interleukin (IL)-12, which triggers the development of T_H1 immunity. Microbe-induced programming might further involve epigenetic modifications at immune-related genes, including histone acetylation.[12]

THE GUT MICROBIOTA AND THE DEVELOPMENT OF ATOPIC DISEASE

The largest collection of human bacteria, by far, is found in the distal gut, consisting of 500 to 1000 different species, including the phyla Bacteroidetes, Firmicutes, Actinobacteria, Proteobacteria, and Verrucomicrobia. The host immune system has evolved to cope with the massive microbial presence by learning to judge correctly between rejecting or accepting new species and to optimally control retained species. In turn, the gut microbiota has developed strategies to both reinforce resistance against harmful invaders and to avoid rejection by the host. These include boosting of host defense as well as the induction of regulatory mechanisms, including the activation of Tregs. Treg induction seems to be a widespread feature of microbiota colonization.[13] The bacterium *Bacteroides fragilis*, for instance, is able to drive the differentiation of IL-10–secreting Tregs, by producing an unusual capsular polysaccharide A,[10] and members of Clostridia metabolize SCFAs, which can have systemic antiinflammatory effects, through influencing DCs and T-cell responses. Segmented filamentous bacteria (SFB) is an example of the opposite, an organism that is able to promote effector responses through driving T_H1 and T_H17 immunity.[14] SFB has a specific feature of adhering strongly to the epithelium of the ileum and Peyer patches,[15] in contrast to most other members of the microbiota, which remain entrapped in the mucus and have little or no physical contact with host epithelium. This feature facilitates sampling and presentation of SFB antigens to T cells by DCs and likely explains the unusual ability of SFB to influence host immunity. Although SFB-deficient mice lack T_H17-type responses and are susceptible to bacterial infections, it is evident that SFB plays a key role in strengthening the gut barrier.

Several studies underline the importance of the composition of the gut microbiota in early life for proper gut development, immune cell maturation, and resistance to pathogens.[16] Moreover, early-life dysbiosis of the gut microbiota has been linked with an increased risk of chronic inflammatory disorders, including allergies, later in life. The mode of delivery is important, with babies born by cesarean section colonized by more *Staphylococcus*, *Corynebacterium*, and *Propionibacterium* species and fewer Bacteroidetes and Actinobacteria compared with vaginally delivered babies, who are enriched for Clostridia.[17] Cesarean birth is linked to predisposition toward asthma during childhood,[18] and studies show that children with an altered or less diverse gut microbiome composition early in life are more likely to develop asthma.[19–21] Moreover, perturbations of the gut microbiome, such as colonization by *Clostridium difficile* at an early age, is significantly associated with the development of wheeze, and recurrent antibiotics, having an impact on on the diversity of the microbiota early in life,[22] correlate with the development of asthma.[23] In contrast, breastfeeding is inversely related with the risk of developing of asthma,[24] and exposure to environmental microbes or farming environments has been associated with protection against asthma.[25–27] It remains to be seen, however, whether the latter also is linked to shifts in communities in the intestines, and whether the gut microbiota can directly drive atopic disease or confer protection against disease remains unclear.

THE CUTANEOUS MICROBIOME AND ATOPIC ECZEMA

The skin is colonized by trillions of microorganisms at a density of 1×10^6 microbes per square millimeter. The composition of the skin microbiota is dependent on the physiology of the site, with sebaceous sites dominated by lipophilic organisms, such as *Propionibacterium* species, and humid environments inhabited mainly by *Staphylococcus* and *Corynebacterium* species.[28] Skin communities are stable over time, especially in the more sheltered areas, despite external challenges, such as sudden changes in temperature, windiness, humidity, clothing, sweating, or the use of skin products. Studies have shown that this stability is dependent on the maintenance of species and strains over time rather than on the acquisition of species from the environment.[29] Compared with the gut, the skin is a hostile environment to microbes—scarce in nutrients, high in salt concentration and antimicrobial peptides, and endowed with a low pH.[30] Nevertheless, a few phyla have adapted well to these conditions, including Actinobacteria, Bacteroidetes, Firmicutes and Proteobacteria—which also are abundantly present in the gut, but at different proportions compared with the skin.

Similar to the gut microbiota, the skin microbiota is essential in the protection against invaders and in educating the skin immune system as well as in skin metabolism and xenometabolism.[31] Skin microbes contribute to the maintenance of a physical and immune barrier of the host and are able to induce the production of antimicrobial peptides and activate complement, and regulate the levels of IL-β produced by keratinocytes and local antigen-presenting cells (APCs), which in turn control the capacity of resident T cells to produce IL-17 and interferon-γ.[32] Thus, analogous to the gut microbiota, skin microorganisms can act as adjuvants to the skin immune system.

One of the functions of normal skin microbiota is to suppress the growth of the pathogen *Staphylococcus aureus*, utilizing several mechanisms. For instance, *S epidermidis* can generate peptide antibiotics (lantibiotics) with bactericidal effects against *S aureus*. Moreover, a lantibiotic produced by *S hominis*, can act synergistically with host antimicrobial peptides. *S epidermidis* also is able to release phenol-soluble modulins, which specifically inhibit *S aureus* and act cooperatively with host antimicrobial peptides. Moreover, *Propionibacterium acnes* may inhibit the growth of *S aureus*, through the generation of fatty acids by fermenting glycerol in sebum, which lowers the local pH in skin.[33] These bacteria are common on healthy skin but typically lacking in inflamed skin, especially in AD.

Whether the microbiota is able to induce antiinflammatory responses in the skin remains unclear. Skin contains the highest frequencies of Tregs in the body, and a large fraction of these can be found in the vicinity of hair follicles.[34] In neonates, but not in adults, the colonization by *S epidermidis* results in an influx of activated Tregs, and blocking their entry prevents tolerance to commensals.[35] Tregs play an important role in calibrating the immune response to microorganisms, but, although the skin microbiota continuously undergoes shifts defined by developmental stages and in the context of disease and infections, it remains unknown how the responses to these microbial fluctuations are controlled. There are some examples of skin commensals that promote regulatory responses, including *Vitreoscilla filiformis*, originally found in thermal spa water, which can promote the accumulation of Tregs in the skin and protect against AD.[36] Moreover, *S epidermidis* is known to induce IL-10 production by DC in vitro,[37] and *Acinetobacter lwoffii* is able to promote both IL-10 production and T_H1 responses in the skin, conferring systemic protection against allergic sensitization and inflammation in a mouse model.[38]

AD is a chronic inflammatory skin disease, characterized by intense itch and recurrent, inflammatory eczematous lesions.[39] AD is one of the most common chronic diseases and affects up to one-fifth of the population in developed countries. Previously, AD pathogenesis was believed to be mediated primarily by abnormalities of humoral and T-cell–mediated immunity, but recently, the epidermis and its barrier functions have been placed at the forefront of research and management efforts. The strongest risk factor of AD is a positive family history for atopic diseases,[40] and systematic gene mapping studies have identified multiple risk loci for AD. For instance, mutations in the filaggrin gene (FLG) gene, which is involved in the formation of the epidermal skin barrier, have been identified as major predisposing factors for atopic eczema.[41] The, to date, approximately 30 identified susceptibility loci, however, explain less than 20% of the estimated heritability. For instance, most patients with AD do not have any FLG mutations, and up to 60% of FLG mutation carriers do not develop atopic disease. Many of the risk genes contribute to immune abnormalities, in particular innate immune signaling and T-cell activation. Most of them also are linked, however, to other inflammatory diseases, suggesting that atopy nonspecific processes are involved. Instead, environmental factors, such as the living environment, lifestyle, and diet, are believed to drive the inherited disease susceptibility predisposition into manifestation. Although the incidence of AD has increased by 2-fold to 3-fold during the past decades in industrialized countries,[42] it has been suggested that a westernized lifestyle may influence the disease outcome. Few proposed environmental risks are supported, however, by strong epidemiologic data, and, in general, little is known about how inherited and environmental factors interact and how this pertains to disease pathophysiology, course, and outcomes.

The skin microbiota frequently is disrupted in AD, with the diversity of the microbiota greatly reduced in favor of the genus *Staphylococcus* — *S aureus*, in particular. AD is a chronic, relapsing condition, with shifts in the microbiota associated with disease flares.[43] *S aureus* is an established trigger to disease,[44] but how the skin microbiota modulates disease is poorly understood. Treatment with antibiotics often is successful, with decreasing disease severity along with the reduction of *S aureus* abundance.[45] S aureus is known to express several molecules, which may contribute to the intensity of the symptoms, including delta toxin, which stimulates mast cells, and alpha toxin, which damages the skin barrier through destroying keratinocytes. S aureus also is able to generate phenol-soluble modulins, which stimulate cytokine release; proteases, which damage the epidermal barrier; and superantigens, which give rise to specific IgE and exacerbate the inflammatory response through nonspecific activation of T cells.[46,47] Recent studies reveal specific differences between staphylococcal strains in the capacity to elicit skin inflammation, and certain strains are particularly able and better suited than others at colonizing the inflammatory skin site in AD skin,[48,49] which contributes to the complexity of AD.

It remains unknown which host or microbiome-derived mechanisms either promote or inhibit the colonization of AD skin by S aureus and what the conditions are that trigger changes to the skin microbiota at the beginning of an AD flare. S. aureus usually dominates the bacterial skin community in AD, along with an extensive loss of other potentially beneficial species of bacteria. These bacteria may contribute to a healthy skin environment through the generation of short chain fatty acids, which may function both as relevant natural moisturizing factors and through lowering the skin pH.[33] Moreover, certain gram positive anaerobic cocci (GPACs), including Finegoldia, stimulate rapid induction of antimicrobial peptides in human keratinocytes, constituting an important signalling mechanism to the keratinocytes when the skin is injured.[50] Therefore, the complete or partial absence of these potentially beneficial microbes may exacerbate a dry and alkaline skin surface environment, and may cause impaired danger signalling in the skin, priming it for further pathogen growth and inflammation.

THE RESPIRATORY MICROBIOME AND ASTHMA

Until recently, the lung has been considered a sterile organ lacking microbial inhabitants. Now, however, it has become evident that the healthy respiratory mucosa is colonized by a range of bacterial communities.[51] The relative abundance and load of these phyla differ significantly from that of other body compartments, with the lower respiratory tract among the least populated surfaces of the human body, with an estimated number of 10 to 100 bacteria per 1000 human cells. The 2 predominant phyla in the airways are Firmicutes and Bacteroidetes, with Actinobacteria, Proteobacteria, and Fusobacteria minor constituents of the local microbiota. Like elsewhere on mucosal surfaces, a balance between immune tolerance and inflammation must be maintained in the lung and is in part regulated by the cross-talk between immune cells and the microbiome.[52] Changes in the microbial composition may negatively influence the immune homeostatic networks, which has been clearly demonstrated in germ-free mice, which display impaired tolerance and increased susceptibility to inflammation or infections.[53] Likely there is substantial cross-talk between mucosal sites, in particular the lung and the gut, because chronic lung disorders often exhibit intestinal disease manifestation, and, conversely, respiratory infections often are accompanied by intestinal indications.[54]

The composition of the airway microbiota develops extensively from the time point of birth and is influenced by the environment. Although it is clear that the microbiome significantly influences host immune maturation and activity, it remains unclear to what extent patterns of airway microbial dysbiosis actually drives disease. Birth mode (vaginal or cesarean section) greatly influences the development of the gut, skin, and respiratory microbiota, with implications for health later on, and the exposure to environments conferred with a high microbial burden and diversity have proved to influence the risk of developing atopic disease and asthma.[26,55]

Mouse models clearly show that the microbiome has a role in the development of airway diseases. One study has shown that the susceptibility to house dust mite (HDM)-induced lung inflammation in a mouse model is dependent on age and associated with the gradually increasing load of Bacteroidetes in the lung. The younger mice that were exposed to HDM generated significantly more exaggerated T_H2-type responses compared with older mice.[56] The protective effect in the older mice was associated with an increased number of bacteria in the airways and a shift from predominance of Gammaproteobacteria and Firmicutes to Bacteroidetes. Oral supplementation of beneficial microbes, such as Bifidobacterium, or microbial metabolites, such as SCFAs, similarly has provided protection against allergic sensitization and inflammation, providing evidence that the gut and lung are closely linked in this context. Several studies also have suggested that direct exposure of the respiratory epithelium to microbial products provides some protective effects. For instance, exposure to dust from farm environments protects mice against HDM-induced asthma via A20-dependent mechanisms in the airway epithelium.[55] Furthermore, Stein and colleagues[26] have shown that exposure of mice via the airways to dust from Amish houses, but not Hutterite houses, protect against asthma in mice, via MyD88-dependent and Trif-dependent mechanisms.

In humans, the risk of asthma is associated with lifestyle and microbial exposures, and early-life dysbiosis of the gut microbiota has been consistently associated with the increased risk of asthma later in life. Asthma recently has been shown to associate also with a significant dysbiosis in the airway microbiota, including an increase in the diversity the phylum Proteobacteria,[57] with the appearance of families, such as Comamonadaceae, Sphingomonadaceae, and Pseudomonadaceae. These results are still controversial, however, and further clinical trials and microbiome studies are needed.

THE KARELIA STUDY

In the author's study, focusing on children in Finnish and Russian Karelia, allergic symptoms and atopic diseases are systematically more common in Finnish children and adults compared with their Russian counterparts. These 2 adjacent areas are geologically and climatically similar but socioeconomically highly distinct. In Russian Karelia, hay fever is almost nonexistent, and only 2% of the children are sensitized to birch pollen. In Finland, approximately one-sixth of the children suffer from hay fever, and 27% are sensitized to birch pollen.[58] On the Finnish side, the author showed that biodiversity of the living environment is related to the composition of the microbiota on the skin in these children and the risk of developing allergic disease. Furthermore, the author observed that the abundance on the skin of the phylum Gammaproteobacteria down to the genus-level Acinetobacter in these children was significantly associated with the capacity of the immune cells in peripheral blood to produce antiinflammatory cytokine IL-10,[25] feeding into a network of regulatory gene expression. The author further examined the capacity of Acinetobacter to modify immune responses in vitro and in vivo and found that compared with other human commensals, including S epidermidis and E. coli, Acinetobacter species were particularly potent at inducing antiinflammatory and T_H1-type immune responses in human keratinocytes and human monocyte–derived DCs as well as locally in the skin in a mouse model, protecting against systemic allergic sensitization and inflammation.[38] Both the diversity and the abundance of Acinetobacter species on the skin and on the nasal epithelium were significantly higher in Russian children compared with children in Finnish Karelia, linking cutaneous Acinetobacter with the unusually low prevalence of allergic disease in the Russian area.[59]

Finally, to establish causality between exposure to environmental biodiversity and the tuning of host microbiomes and the immune system, the author exposed mice to soil for 2.5 months, using siblings kept on clean bedding as controls. Exposure to soil modified the gut microbiota of the mice extensively, including a significant shift in its composition including an increased abundance of Bacteroidetes relative to Firmicutes. A low ratio of Bacteroidetes to Firmicutes in the gut microbiota previously was linked by several studies to various inflammatory conditions, such as obesity[60] and diabetes[61] and the development of asthma in human babies.[62,63] Moreover, in the soil exposed mice, the author observed significantly up-regulated expression of antiinflammatory signaling in the intestinal epithelium of the ileum, which is the most distal part of the small intestines. The ileum is an immunologically highly active tissue, containing numerous Peyer patches, which are engaged in the surveillance of microorganisms in the intestinal lumen and facilitate the generation of immune responses within the mucosa.[64] When exposing the mice to the experimental asthma protocol, the author observed that the inflammatory response was significantly alleviated in the soil exposed mice.[27] Thus, the author's work provides evidence of the role of environmentally acquired microbes in modifying the gut microbiota, and alleviating T_H2-driven allergic inflammation.

SUMMARY

The living environment has profound influence on human health, mediated in part by modifications in the human microbiota. The human microbiota in turn influences both the development and the calibration of the immune system, with consequences for human health. The prevalence of allergies has reached epidemic levels during the past 4 decades, especially in high-income countries, and there is evidence that this phenomenon might be linked to reduced exposures to beneficial environmental microorganisms, and allergic disease often is associated with perturbations in the human microbiota. It remains unclear, however, if microbial dysbiosis actually can drive relevant disease mechanisms or if it simply reflects associated phenomena, such as altered patterns of immune responses to microbes and environmental stimuli.

REFERENCES

1. Ochman H, Worobey M, Kuo CH, et al. Evolutionary relationships of wild hominids recapitulated by gut microbial communities. PLoS Biol 2010;8:e1000546.
2. Wikoff WR, Anfora AT, Liu J, et al. Metabolomics analysis reveals large effects of gut microflora on mammalian blood metabolites. Proc Natl Acad Sci U S A 2009; 106:3698–703.
3. Bogaert D, Keijser B, Huse S, et al. Variability and diversity of nasopharyngeal microbiota in children: a metagenomic analysis. PLoS One 2011;6:e17035.
4. Ravel J, Gajer P, Abdo Z, et al. Vaginal microbiome of reproductive-age women. Proc Natl Acad Sci U S A 2011;108(Suppl 1):4680–7.
5. Blaser MJ. Who are we? Indigenous microbes and the ecology of human diseases. EMBO Rep 2006;7:956–60.
6. Strachan DP. Hay fever, hygiene, and household size. BMJ 1989;299:1259–60.
7. Rook GA. 99th Dahlem conference on infection, inflammation and chronic inflammatory disorders: darwinian medicine and the 'hygiene' or 'old friends' hypothesis. Clin Exp Immunol 2010;160:70–9.
8. von Hertzen L, Hanski I, Haahtela T. Natural immunity. Biodiversity loss and inflammatory diseases are two global megatrends that might be related. EMBO Rep 2011;12:1089–93.

9. Rook GA, Raison CL, Lowry CA. Microbial "Old Friends", immunoregulation and socio-economic status. Clin Exp Immunol 2014;177(1):1–12.

10. Round JL, Mazmanian SK. Inducible Foxp3+ regulatory T-cell development by a commensal bacterium of the intestinal microbiota. Proc Natl Acad Sci U S A 2010; 107:12204–9.

11. Atarashi K, Tanoue T, Oshima K, et al. Treg induction by a rationally selected mixture of Clostridia strains from the human microbiota. Nature 2013;500:232–6.

12. Brand S, Teich R, Dicke T, et al. Epigenetic regulation in murine offspring as a novel mechanism for transmaternal asthma protection induced by microbes. J Allergy Clin Immunol 2011;128:618–25.e1-7.

13. Geuking MB, Cahenzli J, Lawson MA, et al. Intestinal bacterial colonization induces mutualistic regulatory T cell responses. Immunity 2011;34:794–806.

14. Ivanov II, Atarashi K, Manel N, et al. Induction of intestinal Th17 cells by segmented filamentous bacteria. Cell 2009;139:485–98.

15. Klaasen HL, Koopman JP, Van den Brink ME, et al. Intestinal, segmented, filamentous bacteria in a wide range of vertebrate species. Lab Anim 1993;27: 141–50.

16. Sommer F, Backhed F. The gut microbiota–masters of host development and physiology. Nat Rev Microbiol 2013;11:227–38.

17. Rusconi F, Zugna D, Annesi-Maesano I, et al. Mode of delivery and asthma at school age in 9 European Birth Cohorts. Am J Epidemiol 2017;185:465–73.

18. Thavagnanam S, Fleming J, Bromley A, et al. A meta-analysis of the association between Caesarean section and childhood asthma. Clin Exp Allergy 2008;38: 629–33.

19. Stokholm J, Blaser MJ, Thorsen J, et al. Maturation of the gut microbiome and risk of asthma in childhood. Nat Commun 2018;9:141.

20. Abrahamsson TR, Jakobsson HE, Andersson AF, et al. Low gut microbiota diversity in early infancy precedes asthma at school age. Clin Exp Allergy 2014;44: 842–50.

21. Bisgaard H, Li N, Bonnelykke K, et al. Reduced diversity of the intestinal microbiota during infancy is associated with increased risk of allergic disease at school age. J Allergy Clin Immunol 2011;128:646–52.e1-5.

22. Fouhy F, Guinane CM, Hussey S, et al. High-throughput sequencing reveals the incomplete, short-term recovery of infant gut microbiota following parenteral antibiotic treatment with ampicillin and gentamicin. Antimicrob Agents Chemother 2012;56:5811–20.

23. Fanaro S, Chierici R, Guerrini P, et al. Intestinal microflora in early infancy: composition and development. Acta Paediatr Suppl 2003;91:48–55.

24. Kull I, Almqvist C, Lilja G, et al. Breast-feeding reduces the risk of asthma during the first 4 years of life. J Allergy Clin Immunol 2004;114:755–60.

25. Hanski I, von Hertzen L, Fyhrquist N, et al. Environmental biodiversity, human microbiota, and allergy are interrelated. Proc Natl Acad Sci U S A 2012;109:8334–9.

26. Stein MM, Hrusch CL, Gozdz J, et al. Innate immunity and asthma risk in Amish and Hutterite farm children. N Engl J Med 2016;375:411–21.

27. Ottman N, Ruokolainen L, Suomalainen A, et al. Soil exposure modifies the gut microbiota and supports immune tolerance in a mouse model. J Allergy Clin Immunol 2019;143(3):1198–206.e12.

28. Byrd AL, Belkaid Y, Segre JA. The human skin microbiome. Nat Rev Microbiol 2018;16:143–55.

29. Oh J, Byrd AL, Park M, et al. Temporal stability of the human skin microbiome. Cell 2016;165:854–66.

30. Fyhrquist N, Salava A, Auvinen P, et al. Skin Biomes. Curr Allergy Asthma Rep 2016;16:40.
31. Belkaid Y, Tamoutounour S. The influence of skin microorganisms on cutaneous immunity. Nat Rev Immunol 2016;16:353–66.
32. Belkaid Y, Segre JA. Dialogue between skin microbiota and immunity. Science 2014;346:954–9.
33. Panther DJ, Jacob SE. The importance of acidification in atopic eczema: an underexplored avenue for treatment. J Clin Med 2015;4:970–8.
34. Sanchez Rodriguez R, Pauli ML, Neuhaus IM, et al. Memory regulatory T cells reside in human skin. J Clin Invest 2014;124:1027–36.
35. Scharschmidt TC, Vasquez KS, Truong HA, et al. A wave of regulatory t cells into neonatal skin mediates tolerance to commensal microbes. Immunity 2015;43: 1011–21.
36. Volz T, Skabytska Y, Guenova E, et al. Nonpathogenic bacteria alleviating atopic dermatitis inflammation induce IL-10-producing dendritic cells and regulatory Tr1 cells. J Invest Dermatol 2014;134:96–104.
37. Laborel-Preneron E, Bianchi P, Boralevi F, et al. Effects of the Staphylococcus aureus and Staphylococcus epidermidis secretomes isolated from the skin microbiota of atopic children on CD4+ T cell activation. PLoS One 2015;10: e0141067.
38. Fyhrquist N, Ruokolainen L, Suomalainen A, et al. Acinetobacter species in the skin microbiota protect against allergic sensitization and inflammation. J Allergy Clin Immunol 2014;134:1301–9.e11.
39. Weidinger S, Novak N. Atopic dermatitis. Lancet 2016;387:1109–22.
40. Apfelbacher CJ, Diepgen TL, Schmitt J. Determinants of eczema: population-based cross-sectional study in Germany. Allergy 2011;66:206–13.
41. Akiyama M. FLG mutations in ichthyosis vulgaris and atopic eczema: spectrum of mutations and population genetics. Br J Dermatol 2010;162:472–7.
42. Nutten S. Atopic dermatitis: global epidemiology and risk factors. Ann Nutr Metab 2015;66(Suppl 1):8–16.
43. Kong HH, Oh J, Deming C, et al. Temporal shifts in the skin microbiome associated with disease flares and treatment in children with atopic dermatitis. Genome Res 2012;22:850–9.
44. Leyden JJ, Marples RR, Kligman AM. Staphylococcus aureus in the lesions of atopic dermatitis. Br J Dermatol 1974;90:525–30.
45. Huang JT, Abrams M, Tlougan B, et al. Treatment of Staphylococcus aureus colonization in atopic dermatitis decreases disease severity. Pediatrics 2009;123: e808–14.
46. Savinko T, Lauerma A, Lehtimäki S, et al. Topical superantigen exposure induces epidermal accumulation of CD8+ T cells, a mixed Th1/Th2-type dermatitis and vigorous production of IgE antibodies in the murine model of atopic dermatitis. J Immunol 2005;175:8320–6.
47. Wickersham M, Wachtel S, Wong Fok Lung T, et al. Metabolic stress drives keratinocyte defenses against Staphylococcus aureus infection. Cell Rep 2017;18: 2742–51.
48. Byrd AL, Deming C, Cassidy SKB, et al. Staphylococcus aureus and Staphylococcus epidermidis strain diversity underlying pediatric atopic dermatitis. Sci Transl Med 2017;9 [pii:eaal4651].
49. Yeung M, Balma-Mena A, Shear N, et al. Identification of major clonal complexes and toxin producing strains among Staphylococcus aureus associated with atopic dermatitis. Microbes Infect 2011;13:189–97.

50. Zeeuwen PL, Ederveen TH, van der Krieken DA, et al. Gram-positive anaerobe cocci are underrepresented in the microbiome of filaggrin-deficient human skin. J Allergy Clin Immunol 2017;139:1368–71.
51. Denner DR, Sangwan N, Becker JB, et al. Corticosteroid therapy and airflow obstruction influence the bronchial microbiome, which is distinct from that of bronchoalveolar lavage in asthmatic airways. J Allergy Clin Immunol 2016;137: 1398–405.e3.
52. Frei R, Lauener RP, Crameri R, et al. Microbiota and dietary interactions: an update to the hygiene hypothesis? Allergy 2012;67:451–61.
53. Herbst T, Sichelstiel A, Schär C, et al. Dysregulation of allergic airway inflammation in the absence of microbial colonization. Am J Respir Crit Care Med 2011; 184:198–205.
54. Marsland BJ, Trompette A, Gollwitzer ES. The gut-lung axis in respiratory disease. Ann Am Thorac Soc 2015;12(Suppl 2):S150–6.
55. Schuijs MJ, Willart MA, Vergote K, et al. Farm dust and endotoxin protect against allergy through A20 induction in lung epithelial cells. Science 2015;349:1106–10.
56. Gollwitzer ES, Saglani S, Trompette A, et al. Lung microbiota promotes tolerance to allergens in neonates via PD-L1. Nat Med 2014;20:642–7.
57. Huang YJ, Nelson CE, Brodie EL, et al. Airway microbiota and bronchial hyperresponsiveness in patients with suboptimally controlled asthma. J Allergy Clin Immunol 2011;127:372–81.e1-3.
58. Haahtela T, Laatikainen T, Alenius H, et al. Hunt for the origin of allergy - comparing the Finnish and Russian Karelia. Clin Exp Allergy 2015;45:891–901.
59. Ruokolainen L, Paalanen L, Karkman A, et al. Significant disparities in allergy prevalence and microbiota between the young people in Finnish and Russian Karelia. Clin Exp Allergy 2017;47:665–74.
60. Turnbaugh PJ, Ley RE, Mahowald MA, et al. An obesity-associated gut microbiome with increased capacity for energy harvest. Nature 2006;444:1027–31.
61. Roesch LF, Lorca GL, Casella G, et al. Culture-independent identification of gut bacteria correlated with the onset of diabetes in a rat model. ISME J 2009;3(5): 536–48.
62. Thorburn AN, McKenzie CI, Shen S, et al. Evidence that asthma is a developmental origin disease influenced by maternal diet and bacterial metabolites. Nat Commun 2015;6:7320.
63. Trompette A, Gollwitzer ES, Yadava K, et al. Gut microbiota metabolism of dietary fiber influences allergic airway disease and hematopoiesis. Nat Med 2014;20(2): 159–66.
64. Lelouard H, Fallet M, de Bovis B, et al. Peyer's patch dendritic cells sample antigens by extending dendrites through M cell-specific transcellular pores. Gastroenterology 2012;142:592–601.e3.

Mood and Microbes
Gut to Brain Communication in Depression

John R. Kelly, MD, PhD[a], Veronica O' Keane, MD, PhD[a],
John F. Cryan, PhD[b,c], Gerard Clarke, PhD[b,d],
Timothy G. Dinan, MD, PhD[b,d],*

KEYWORDS

- Microbiota • Microbiome • Gut-brain axis • Immune system • Depression • Anxiety
- Psychobiotics

KEY POINTS

- Converging preclinical data show that a complex network of lifelong microbial signaling pathways from gut to brain mediates many of the domains dysregulated in depression.
- Altered gut microbiota profiles have been demonstrated in depressed patients.
- Fecal microbiota transfer studies using germ free and microbiota-depleted rodents, suggest that the gut microbiota plays a physiological role in depression.
- Antidepressant and antipsychotic medication can impact the gut microbiota, but the implications of this drug–gut microbiota interaction are not fully known.
- Well-powered, prospective, interventional clinical studies, of psychobiotic strategies (probiotics, prebiotics, diet) with central markers of brain function, are required to ascertain whether the gut microbiota and its metabolic output will serve as useful biosignatures to advance personalized precision treatment or preventive strategies in psychiatry.

Disclosure Statement: The APC Microbiome Institute is funded by Science Foundation Ireland (SFI). This publication has emanated from research conducted with the financial support of SFI under grant SFI/12/RC/2273. The authors and their work were also supported by the Health Research Board through Health Research Awards (grants HRA_POR/2011/23: T.G. Dinan, J.F. Cryan, and G. Clarke; HRA_POR/2012/32: J.F. Cryan, T.G. Dinan, and HRA-POR-2-14-647: G. Clarke, T.G. Dinan) and through EUGRANT613979 (MYNEWGUTFP7-KBBE-2013-7). The center has conducted studies in collaboration with several companies, including GSK, Pfizer, Wyeth, and Mead Johnson. G. Clarke is supported by an NARSAD Young Investigator Grant from the Brain and Behavior Research Foundation (grant 20771).

[a] Department of Psychiatry, Trinity College Dublin and Tallaght Hospital, Trinity Centre for Health Sciences, Tallaght University Hospital, Dublin 24, Ireland; [b] APC Microbiome Ireland, University College Cork, Cork, Ireland; [c] Department of Anatomy and Neuroscience, University College Cork, Room 2,33, 2nd Floor, Western Gateway Building, Cork, Ireland; [d] Department of Psychiatry and Neurobehavioral Science, Biosciences Institute, University College Cork, College Road, Cork, Ireland
* Corresponding author.
E-mail address: t.dinan@ucc.ie

Gastroenterol Clin N Am 48 (2019) 389–405
https://doi.org/10.1016/j.gtc.2019.04.006

INTRODUCTION

There is a growing recognition of the role played by gut microbes in human health. The extension of this role, to encompass brain health, has come into focus in recent years. Microbes, by recruiting the bidirectional communication network of the gut-brain axis, exert an influence over many of the processes involved in brain development and function.[1,2] Although the precise mechanisms have yet to be fully elucidated, there are several putative mechanisms by which the gut microbiota can influence brain development and function; via modulation of the immune system,[3] the hypothalamic-pituitary-adrenal (HPA) axis,[4] tryptophan metabolism,[5] the production of bacterial metabolites, such as short chain fatty acids (SCFAs),[6] via the vagus nerve[7] and via bacterial peptidoglycan.[8] Many of these pathways are of direct relevance to neuropsychiatric disorders.

Depression, commonly comorbid with anxiety, is a complex, heterogeneous, predominately recurrent disorder that leads to significant levels of disability worldwide.[9] The neurobiological underpinnings of depression involve dysregulated neuro-immune and neuro-endocrine systems, in addition to deficits in synaptic plasticity, impaired neurogenesis, and reduced hippocampal volumes. There is an increasing need to elucidate the interaction of biological and environmental processes at an integrative mechanistic level in neuropsychiatric disorders. Preliminary attempts at biomarker development have been attempted, although none have translated to the clinic. Indeed, a single approach to uncovering the mechanistic complexities underlying neuropsychiatric disorders, such as depression and anxiety, is likely to be insufficient.

Clinicians treat patients by a trial and error approach, leading to delays in response and remission. The need to progress precision psychiatry, based on underlying biological mechanisms, to assist clinicians in making treatment choices based on biosignatures is crucial. Exploration of the gut microbiota and its influence over the molecular substrates defective in neuropsychiatric domains, offers an opportunity to advance this process, and in conjunction with other biomarkers may ultimately lead to treatment or preventive strategies.[10] Here, we review the neurobiological systems of relevance to neuropsychiatric disorders that are under the influence of the gut microbiota, with particular focus on depression and anxiety.

MICROBIOTA AND STRESS

Stress can impact the gut microbiota and reshape its composition, affecting the regulation of the proinflammatory cytokine interleukin (IL)-6,[11] peripheral components of the HPA axis, and local metabolism of glucocorticoids.[12] Early-life is a particularly vulnerable period for the subsequent emergence of neuropsychiatric disorders in adulthood. Preclinical evidence suggests that the gut microbiota signature acquired and nurtured during this pivotal early-life stage may influence stress reactivity.[13] Germ free (GF) rodents demonstrate abnormal behavioral and neuroendocrine responses to stress.[4] Moreover, the normal development of the HPA axis is contingent on microbiota colonization at specific neurodevelopmental time points.[4] The expression of anxiety-like behavior in a mouse model of early-life stress has been shown to be partially dependent on the gut microbiota.[14] Interestingly, a diet consisting of prebiotics and *Lactobacillus rhamnonsus* GG attenuated the anxietylike behavioral effects of early-life maternal separation and deficits in hippocampal-dependent learning in mice.[15]

Prenatal stress also impacts the gut microbiota with implications for physiologic outcomes in the offspring.[16] In a mouse model of prenatal stress, maternal stress decreased the abundance of vaginal *Lactobacillus*, resulting in decreased transmission of this bacterium to offspring, which corresponded with changes in metabolite profiles involved in energy balance, and with disruptions of amino acid profiles in the developing brain.[17] The same research group highlighted the importance of the vaginal microbiome in the stress response system. They demonstrated that transplantation of maternal vaginal microbiota from stressed dams into naive pups delivered by C-section had effects that partly resembled those seen in prenatally stressed males.[18] Moreover, the maternal vaginal transfer also partially mediated the effects of prenatal stress on hypothalamic gene expression.[18] Human infants of mothers with high self-reported stress and high salivary cortisol concentrations during pregnancy had significantly higher relative abundances of Proteobacteria groups known to contain pathogens and lower relative abundances of lactic acid bacteria (*Lactobacillus*) and *Bifidobacteria*.[19]

MICROBIOTA AND THE IMMUNE SYSTEM

The immune system and the central nervous system (CNS) are in constant dialogue. Neuroimmune signaling during the prenatal or early postnatal developmental stages can have long-lasting effects on the brain, and is an important determinant of emotional behavior and cognitive function. A critical function of the gut microbiota is to prime the development of the neuroimmune system. The "old friends hypothesis" proposes that encountering less microbial biodiversity may contribute to an increase in chronic inflammatory disorders, including depression,[20] whereas a more diverse microbial biodiversity, especially during specific vulnerable neurodevelopmental periods, may promote resilience.[21] A compelling strategy of "reintroducing" old friends, has been suggested by a preclinical study using heat-killed *Mycobacterium vaccae*, an immunoregulatory environmental microorganism. Mice given this vaccine exhibited reduced subordinate, flight, and avoiding behavioral responses to a dominant aggressor in a model of chronic psychosocial stress compared with the control group.[22] Depletion of regulatory T cells negated the protective effects of immunization with *M. vaccae* on anxiety-like or fear behaviors.[22] *M. vaccae* also prevented stress-induced priming of the microglia proinflammatory response,[23] altered subsets of serotonergic neurons in the brainstem, and induced antidepressant-like behavioral responses.[24,25]

Microglia

Microglia are phagocytic innate immune cells that play a key role in brain development, plasticity, and cognition. Stress results in microglia activation and increased levels of proinflammatory cytokines in areas such as the hippocampus, hypothalamus, and prefrontal cortex.[26] The concept of microglia priming may be of relevance to psychiatric disorders, which often require multiple "hits," especially during sensitive neurodevelopmental windows. It has recently been proposed that the microbiota, by mediating the effects of both prenatal and postnatal factors, in the context of host genetics, may act as a fourth "hit" that interacts with the other factors to program for brain health and disease in later life.[27]

The gut microbiota plays a role in the maturation and activation of microglia.[3] GF mice display underdeveloped and immature microglia in the cortex, corpus callosum, hippocampus, olfactory bulb, and cerebellum.[3] There was an upregulation of microglia transcription and survival factors, and downregulation of cell activation genes and genes for type 1 interferon receptor signaling compared with those isolated from conventionally colonized control mice. These defects were partially restored by recolonization with a complex microbiota, and SCFAs reversed the defective microglia in absence of a complex microbiota.[3] Collectively, these studies suggest that subtle alterations in gut microbiota acquisition and development, by regulating neuro-inflammatory processes may act as additional vulnerability factors that may predispose to neuropsychiatric symptoms.

SEROTONIN AND KYNURENINE

Serotonin (5-HT), and its precursor tryptophan, are signaling molecules in the brain-gut-microbiota axis.[5] Emerging evidence also suggests that the serotonergic system may be under the influence of gut microbiota, especially, but not limited to, periods before the emergence of a stable adultlike gut microbiota.[28,29] For example, colonic tryptophan hydroxylase 1 (Tph1) messenger RNA and protein were increased in humanized GF and conventionally raised mice.[30] Bacterial metabolites also have been demonstrated to influence Tph1 transcription in a human enterochromaffin cell model.[30] Others have demonstrated that distinct microbial metabolites produced by spore-forming bacteria increase colonic and blood 5-HT in chromaffin cell cultures.[31]

The primary route for tryptophan catabolism is via the kynurenine pathway. The enzyme indoleamine 2,3-dioxygenase (IDO), found in macrophages and microglia cells, is the first and rate-limiting step in the kynurenine pathway of tryptophan catabolism. Dysregulation of the kynurenine pathway has implications for depression, as kynurenine can cross the blood brain barrier (BBB) to increase central levels and can result in the production of neurotoxic metabolites.[32] A study in mice using an unpredictable chronic mild stress model, showed decreased *Lactobacillus* levels and increased kynurenine blood levels compared with control mice.[33] Restoration of *Lactobacillus* by the probiotic *Lactobacillus reuteri* was sufficient to improve the metabolic and behavioral abnormalities. Moreover, the investigators identified a *Lactobacillus*-derived reactive oxygen species that suppressed kynurenine metabolism by inhibiting IDO in the intestine.[33]

SHORT CHAIN FATTY ACIDS

SCFAs (butyrate, acetate, and propionate) are neurohormonal signaling molecules produced by certain classes of bacteria. SCFAs can reach the circulation and cross the BBB,[34] and recent studies in GF[35] and antibiotic-treated mice[36] suggest that the BBB may be partially modulated by changes in the gut microbiota. Butyrate also acts as a potent inhibitor of histone deacetylases (HDACs), and as a ligand for a subset of G protein–coupled receptors. This HDAC inhibition has been proposed as a mechanism by which the microbiota via butyrate production acts as a mediator of gene–environment interactions[6]; however, the effects on gene expression in the CNS may be subtle and contingent on cumulative chronic delivery.

Sodium butyrate was shown to have antidepressant-like effects, indicated by reduced immobility time in the tail suspension test in mice, and resulted in histone hyperacetylation in hippocampus and frontal cortex.[37] Chronic administration of sodium butyrate had antidepressant-like effects in rats, measured by the forced swim test (FST), with concomitant alterations in hydroxymethylation of brain-derived neurotrophic factor (BDNF).[38] Conversely, another study in mice showed that acute, but not chronic treatment with sodium butyrate increased immobility time in the FST.[39] In addition, only high doses of sodium butyrate increased markers of stress, such as plasma adrenocorticotrophin hormone, corticosterone, and glucose levels in rats.[40] A recent study in male mice showed that administration of a mixture of acetate, propionate, and butyrate alleviated heightened stress-responsiveness and stress-induced increases in intestinal permeability, while also decreasing anxiety-like behavior in the open field test and decreasing depressive-like behavior in the FST.[41]

GUT MICROBIOTA, FEAR, AND ANXIETY

The neural circuits that underlie fear-related behaviors are complex and depend on functional communication between the amygdala and prefrontal cortex. There is accruing preclinical data to suggest that the microbiota influences amygdala neuronal morphology and function.[42,43] In GF mice, there was upregulation of several immediate early-response genes, such as Fos, Fosb, Egr2, or Nr4a1, in association with increased cyclic AMP response element-binding protein.[44] Moreover, GF mice show attenuated social stimulus–dependent transcriptional regulation in the amygdala, and an increase in expression of splicing factors and exon usage, compared with control mice.[45]

In addition to an altered transcriptional profile in the amygdala, GF mice have recently been shown to exhibit reduced freezing behavior during a cued memory retention test, whereas colonized GF mice were behaviorally comparable to conventionally raised mice during the retention test.[46] MicroRNAs (miRNAs) act through translational repression to control gene translation and have also been implicated in anxietylike behaviors. miRNAs were dysregulated in GF animals in the amygdala and in the prefrontal cortex, and colonization of GF mice normalized some of the alterations.[47]

Dysregulated fear circuits, memory reconsolidation, and fear conditioning are associated with post-traumatic stress disorder (PTSD). In a small exploratory study of subjects with PTSD (n = 18), the relative abundances of *Actinobacteria*, *Lentisphaerae*, and *Verrucomicrobia* were decreased compared with trauma-exposed controls (n = 12). The decreased total abundance of these taxa were associated with higher clinician-administered PTSD scale scores.[48] In a randomized, double-blind, placebo-controlled trial involving healthy human participants (n = 76), the tetracycline antibiotic doxycycline (200 mg), and a matrix metalloproteinase inhibitor, known to alter the composition of the gut microbiota and its metabolomic output, resulted in reduced fear memory retention, measured with fear-potentiated startle 7 days after acquisition compared with participants who received placebo.[49]

MICROBIOTA AND DEPRESSION

Propelled by preclinical studies showing that the gut microbiota can influence many pathways involved in depression, clinical and translational studies investigating the gut microbiota in depression have emerged over recent years (**Table 1**). These exploratory studies show that depression is associated with an altered gut microbiota profile. Furthermore, this altered gut microbiota profile may play a pathophysiological role in depression. Zheng and colleagues[50] showed that GF mice exhibited reduced anxiety-like behavior in the open field test and decreased depressive-like behavior in the FST compared with specific-pathogen-free mice. Fecal microbiota transfer (FMT) from 5 medication-free depressed patients to GF mice, increased depressive and anxiety-like behavior at 2 weeks after FMT compared with mice that received FMT from healthy controls. Shotgun metagenomic analysis on cecal samples showed that several carbohydrate metabolites (α-glucose, β-glucose, fructose, and succinate) were increased in the GF mice that received the depression FMT relative to control mice. This increase in carbohydrate metabolites was also found in fecal, serum, and hippocampal samples, whereas amino acid metabolism dysregulation was evident only in the hippocampus in the mice that received the depression FMT.[50]

Table 1
Microbiota studies in major depressive disorder (MDD)

Design	Diagnosis, n, Age	Measures	Results	Reference
Cross-sectional	MDD (n = 37) Age 42.9 y MADRS: 26.3 Controls (n = 18) Age 46.1 y	16S rRNA (Illumina) 27 MDD on ADTs	MDD: No differences at phylum level ↑ Bacteroidales at order level ↓ Lachnospiraceae at family level ↑Oscillibacter genus, ↑ Alistipes at genus level Diversity: no significant differences in alpha diversity (simpsons), or richness	Naseribafrouei et al,[80] 2014
Cross-sectional	MDD (n = 46) 29 Active Depression (A-MDD): HAMD25 ≥20 Age 25.3 y 17 Responded (R-MDD) Age 27.1 y Controls (n = 18) Age 26.8 y Exclusion: antibiotics, probiotics, prebiotics, or synbiotics in the last month	454 Life Sciences genome sequencer serum cytokines serum BDNF Most prescribed psychotropic medication: 72% (SSRI or SNRI) (A-MDD) 100% (R-MDD) 24% (A-MDD) and 29% (R-MDD) antipsychotics 83% (A-MDD) and 58.9% (R-MDD) benzodiazepines	MDD: Phylum: ↓ Actinobacteria, Firmicutes in a-MDD [relative abundance] ↑ Fusobacteria, Proteobacteria, Bacteroidetes (A-MDD) ↓ Actinobacteria, ªFusobacteria, Firmicutes (R-MDD) ↑ Proteobacteria, Bacteroidetes (R-MDD) MDD: Family: ↓ Veillonellaceae, Prevotellaceae, Lachnospiraceae, Erysipelotrichaceae, Bacteroidaceae (A-MDD) ↑ Rikenellaceae, Porphyromonadaceae, Fusobacteriaceae, Enterobacteriae, Acidaminococcaceae (A-MDD) MDD: Genus: ↓ Veillonellaceae, Ruminoccaceae, Lachnospiraceae (R-MDD) ↑ Bacteroidaceae, Rikenellaceae, Porphyromonadaceae, Enterobacteriae, Acidaminococcaceae (R-MDD) ↓ Ruminococcus, Prevotella, Faecalibacterium, Dialister, Bacteroides (A-MDD)	Jiang et al,[54] 2015

↑ *Roseburia* (Lachnospiraceae family), *Oscillibacter, Phascolarctobacterium, Parabacteroides, Megamonas, Lachnospiracea incertae sedis* (A-MDD)

↑ *Clostridium XIX, Blautia* (Lachnospiraceae family), *Alistipes* (A-MDD)

↓ *Ruminococcus, Prevotella, Faecalibacterium, ᵃDialister, Oscillibacter, Escherichia/Shigella* (R-MDD)

↑ *Bacteroides, Roseburia, Phascolarcto bacterium, Parabacteroides, Alistipes* (R-MDD)

Diversity:

Shannon diversity significantly higher in (A-MDD) vs HC

No significant difference in richness (ACE, Chao1) or evenness

No separation by beta diversity (unweighted UniFrac & PCA)

Relative abundances of *Clostridium XIVb* (genera), negatively correlated with the serum BDNF levels (r = −0.32)

Relative abundances of Faecalibacterium (genera) negatively correlated with severity of depressive symptoms (HAMD) (r = −0.30), & MADRS (r = −0.37)

MDD:

No significant differences in TNF-a, IL-1b, IL-6 levels

BDNF significantly lower in (A-MDD) & (R-MDD) vs HC

(continued on next page)

Table 1
(continued)

Design	Diagnosis, n, Age	Measures	Results	Reference
Cross-sectional/ Translational	58 MDD (39 drug-naïve) 63 controls Lack of detailed dietary information	16S rRNA Adult (6–8/52) male GF Kunming mice OFT, FST, TST Metabolomics: Multiplex shotgun metagenomic analysis (Illumina HiSeq2500) on cecal samples Cecum, serum and hippocampus Gas chromatography–mass spectrometry, liquid chromatography–mass spectrometry & nuclear magnetic resonance	Relative abundances at phylum level: increase in Actinobacteria decrease in Bacteroidetes 29 OTUs were overrepresented in MDD subjects 25 OTUs were overrepresented in healthy control subjects Diversity: No significant differences in alpha diversity Beta diversity; PCoA of unweighted UniFrac, 19% difference between MDD and HC PCoA of weighted UniFrac, 23% difference between MDD and HC Rodent study: 1-wk post FMT: no differences in OFT, FST or TST 2-wk post FMT: increase in immobility time in FST & TST OFT: decreased proportion of central motion distance FST: decreased immobility time MDD FMT: Increase in cecal carbohydrate metabolites (α-glucose, β-glucose, fructose and succinate) (also in fecal, serum samples), hippocampi showed disturbances in carbohydrate metabolism (glucose, lactose and malic acid) and amino acid metabolism (phenylalanine, N-acetyl-L-aspartic acid, glycine and leucine)	Zheng et al,[50] 2016

| Cross-sectional/ Translational | MDD (n = 34)
Age 48 y
Controls (n = 33)
Age 48 y
HAMD 17 (19.5)
majority of depressed patients prescribed ADT | 16S rRNA
Fecal SCFAs
Plasma Inflammatory markers, kynurenine/tryptophan, LBP
Male Sprague-Dawley Rats
Antibiotic-treated model (ampicillin & metronidazole) (all at 1 g/L), vancomycin (500 mg/L), ciprofloxacin HCl (200 mg/L), imipenem (250 mg/L) for 4 wk
FMT - booster inoculations given every 2 wk throughout the 14-wk study | No difference at phylum level
Family level:
MDD:
  ↓ Prevotellaceae
  ↑ Thermoanaerobacteriaceae
Genus level:
  ↑ *Eggerthella, Holdemania, Gelria, Turicibacter, Paraprevotella, Anaerofilum*
  ↓ *Prevotella, Dialister*
MDD:
  ↑ levels of IL-6, IL-8, TNF-a, CRP and kynurenine/tryptophan ratio
  No significant differences in LBP
MDD:
  Chao1 richness, total observed species and phylogenetic diversity decreased
  No difference in Shannon diversity
  No significant differences in fecal SCFAs (acetate, propionate, iso-Butyrate or butyrate)
Rodent study:
  MDD FMT:
    Decrease in sucrose intake in the sucrose preference test
    Decrease in visits to the open arms in the EPM
    Reduction in time spent in the center in OFT
    No difference in FST
    Increase in the plasma Kynurenine/ Tryptophan ratio
  MDD FMT:
    Chao1 & observed species reduced, diversity (phylogenetic diversity and Shannon index) reduced
    Significant differences at the phylum level, the family level and genus level
    Fecal acetate and total SCFAs increased | Kelly et al,[51] 2016 |

(continued on next page)

Table 1
(continued)

Design	Diagnosis, n, Age	Measures	Results	Reference
Interventional Double-blind RCT 8 wk - probiotic containing: L. acidophilus, L. casei and B. bifidum (2*10⁹ CFU/g) added to an SSRI	MDD Probiotic (n = 17) Age 38.3 Placebo (n = 18) Age 36.2 Intention to treat Moderate depression (HAMD-17) Exclusion: probiotics, dietary supplements	Primary outcome: BDI Secondary outcomes: fasting plasma glucose (FPG), markers of insulin metabolism, lipid concentrations, serum high-sensitivity CRP, and biomarkers of oxidative stress, including total antioxidant capacity (TAC) and GSH (total glutathione) Diet & physical activity recorded (3-time points) No gut microbiota analysis	Probiotic group: BDI score decreased Insulin levels decreased HOMA-IR decreased hsCRP decreased Plasma GSH levels increased No significant changes in FPG, Homeostasis model of assessment of B cell function (HOMA-B), Quantitative insulin sensitivity check index (QUICKI), Lipid profiles, TAC levels	Akkasheh et al,[63] 2016
Randomized, double-blind trial for 8 wk Lactobacillus Helveticus and Bifidobacterium longum Medication Free	Probiotic (n = 33) Age 35.8 Placebo (n = 36) Age 35.1 Intention to treat	Clinical measures: MADRS, iCGI, QIDS-SR16, GAF, DASS. Blood markers: CRP, IL-1β, IL-6, TNF-α, BDNF, Vitamin D	No significant difference was found between the probiotic and placebo groups on any psychological outcome measure or any blood-based biomarker At end-point, 9 (23%) of those in the probiotic group showed a ≥60% change on the MADRS (responders), compared to 10 (26%) of those in the placebo group Baseline vitamin D level was found to moderate treatment effect on several outcome measures	Romijn et al,[64] 2017

Abbreviations: ACE, angiotensin-converting enzyme; ADTs, antidepressants; BDI, Beck Depression Inventory; BDNF, brain-derived neurotrophic factor; CRP, C-reactive protein; DASS, Depression Anxiety Stress scale; EPM, elevated plus maze; FMT, fecal microbiota transplantation; FPG, fasting plasma glucose; FST, forced swim test; GAF, global assessment of functioning scale; GSH, total glutathione; HAMD, Hamilton Depression rating scale; HC, health control; HOMA-IR, Homeostasis model of assessment of insulin resistance; hsCRP, high-sensitivity C-reactive protein; iCGI, Improved Clinical Global Impressions scale; IL, interleukin; LBP, Lipopolysaccharide Binding Protein; MADRS, Montgomery–Asberg Depression Rating Scale; MDD, Major Depressive Disorder; OFT, open field test; OTUs, operational taxonomic unit; PCoA, Principal Coordinates Analysis; QIDS-SR16, Quick Inventory of Depressive Symptomatology; RCT, randomized controlled trial; rRNA, ribosomal RNA; SCFAs, short chain fatty acids; SNRI, serotonin–norepinephrine reuptake inhibitor; SSRI, selective serotonin reuptake inhibitor; TAC, total antioxidant capacity; TNF, tumor necrosis factor; TST, tail suspension test; Up arrow, Increase; down arrow, decrease.
[a] Different direction to A-MDD.
Data from Refs.[50,51,54,63,64,80]

We showed that depression is associated with an altered gut microbiota composition including decreased microbial richness and diversity, further suggesting that a diverse gut microbiota may be a health-promoting factor.[51] Using a microbiota-depleted antibiotic rat model, a pooled FMT from 3 of the severely depressed patients induced anhedonia-like behavior, assessed in the sucrose preference test, compared with rats that received the healthy FMT. Furthermore, FMT from the depressed patients induced anxiety-like behaviors, as demonstrated by a significant decrease in visits to the open arms in the elevated plus maze and a reduction in time spent in the center in the open field, compared with rats that received the healthy donor FMT.[51] Dysregulated tryptophan metabolism, as indicated by an increased plasma kynurenine–tryptophan ratio, was demonstrated in both the depressed humans and the rats that received the depression FMT, suggesting that dysregulated tryptophan/kynurenine metabolism is a possible mechanism to account for the depressive and anxiety-like behavior. More recently, a preclinical study using ultra high-performance liquid chromatography–mass spectrometry was performed in a chronic variable stress-induced depression rat model.[52] In this study, there were microbiota differences at the phylum and genus level compared with controls. In addition, there were lower levels of amino acids and fatty acids, and higher amounts of bile acids, hypoxanthine, and stercobilins in the stress-induced group. Moreover, there were substantial associations of perturbed gut microbiota genera with the altered fecal metabolites, especially compounds involved in the metabolism of tryptophan and bile acids.[52]

The first study investigating the gut microbiota in bipolar affective disorder patients (n = 115), showed levels of *Faecalibacterium* were decreased, after adjusting for age, sex, and body mass index, compared with healthy control subjects (n = 64). Moreover, *Faecalibacterium* was associated with better self-reported health outcomes.[53] Interestingly, reduced levels of *Faecalibacterium* were also reported in the study by Jiang and colleagues,[54] which negatively correlated with severity of depressive symptoms. Fecal microbiota signatures in patients with diarrhea-predominant irritable bowel syndrome (IBS), a stress-related gastrointestinal disorder, were shown to be similar to those patients with depression.[55] FMT from patients with IBS to rats induced anxiety-related behaviors in the rats.[56] Collectively, these studies suggest that the gut microbiota may play a pathophysiological role in stress-related disorders.

PSYCHOBIOTICS

Psychobiotics, originally defined as live bacteria that when ingested in adequate amounts can produce a positive mental health benefit, in terms of anxiety, mood, and cognition,[57] have more recently been expanded to encompass "any substance that exerts a microbiome-mediated psychological effect."[58] The process of translating psychobiotics from bench to bedside is not without significant challenges,[59,60] but a growing number of small studies with healthy individuals suggests that prolonged prebiotic and probiotic consumption can positively affect aspects of mood, anxiety, and cognition.[61] Similar to other interventions, probiotic supplements have an individualized impact, in keeping with the advance toward precision-personalized health.[62]

Clinical interventional trials investigating potential psychobiotics in clinical depression are emerging (see **Table 1**). In the first study (n = 40), 8 weeks of a multispecies probiotic containing *Lactobacillus acidophilus, Lactobacillus casei,* and *Bifidobacterium bifidum* added to a selective serotonic reuptake inhibitor, reportedly reduced depressive symptoms in moderately depressed patients compared with placebo.[63] However, the other 8-week double-blind randomized controlled trial (n = 79), conducted in antidepressant-free depressed subjects, failed to show superiority of *actobacillus helveticus* and *Bifidobacterium longum* over placebo.[64] This study should be interpreted with caution, as it recruited participants by self-referral. A recent study suggested that probiotics also may be useful across the mood disorder spectrum. In bipolar affective disorder, patients hospitalized for a manic episode (n = 66) were randomized to receive 24 weeks of adjunctive probiotics (*Lactobacillus rhamnosus strain GG* and *Bifidobacterium animalis* subsp. lactis strain Bb12) or adjunctive placebo at discharge. The probiotic group had lower rates of rehospitalization compared with the group that received the placebo.[65] Several systematic reviews and meta-analyses are emerging. Although limited by analysis of small studies with high levels of heterogeneity, across clinical and nonclinical groups, they mostly corroborate the finding that probiotics can be beneficial in reducing depressive symptoms, although future studies of higher quality and larger sample size are required.

Neuroimaging offers the opportunity to delineate the impact of gut microbiota modulation on brain structure and function. Clinical studies incorporating neuroimaging are beginning to emerge in subjects with IBS. A double-blind randomized controlled trial (n = 44), using functional MRI, showed that 6 weeks of *B longum* NCC3001, attenuated responses to negative emotional stimuli in amygdala and fronto-limbic regions, and reduced depression scores as measured by the Hospital Anxiety and Depression scale compared with placebo.[66] Whereas a structural MRI study in IBS showed that gut microbial composition correlated with sensory and salience-related brain regions.[67] Although preliminary, these studies are beginning to merge microbiome research with neuroimaging to further explore the role of the gut microbiota on neural circuitry.

NUTRITION, THE GUT MICROBIOME AND PSYCHIATRY

Neurodevelopment is contingent on the adequate supply of micronutrients and macronutrients. Many of these nutrients are modulated by the gut microbiota. Omega-3 polyunsaturated fatty acids (ω-3 or n-3 PUFAs), such as eicosapentaenoic acid (EPA) and docosahexaenoic acid (DHA), are essential nutritional compounds for neurodevelopment. Omega-3 supplementation of a high-fat diet increased microbiota diversity and increased *Bifidobacterium* levels in mice.[68] Another study showed that mice supplemented with omega-3 displayed greater fecal *Bifidobacterium* and *Lactobacillus* abundance and dampened HPA-axis activity.[69] A deficit in omega-3 increased depressive-like behavior, impaired communication and social behavior, and affected the metabolome.[70,71]

Diet is one of the most important modifiable determinants of human health that can profoundly alter the composition of the gut microbiota. Indeed, nutritional psychiatry is a nascent field that aims "to develop a comprehensive, cohesive and scientifically rigorous evidence base to support a shift in thinking around the role of diet and nutrition in mental health."[72] Guidelines suggest "traditional" dietary patterns, such as the Mediterranean diet, an increase in consumption of fruits, vegetables, legumes, wholegrain cereals, nuts, and seeds, and inclusion of foods rich in omega-3, can reduce risk of depression.[73]

The Mediterranean diet increased levels of fecal SCFAs, *Prevotella* and some fiber-degrading *Firmicutes*,[74] and it has been suggested that a Mediterranean diet can reduce the incidence of depression.[75] Conversely, a Western diet (processed or fried foods, refined grains, sugary products, and beer) has been associated with depressive symptoms.[76] Interestingly, a recent study showed that a diet of nitrated dry cured meats was associated with manic episodes.[77] Furthermore, reported in the same study a nitrate-supplemented diet fed to rats resulted in hyperactivity and changes in the intestinal microbiota composition.[77]

DRUG–MICROBIOME INTERACTIONS

In recent years, there has been a focus on the complex interaction between the gut microbiota and drug metabolism. Nonantibiotic drugs, including many psychotropic drugs, have a marked impact on the gut microbiota.[78] In a well-powered, cross-sectional microbiome study, medication had the largest explanatory power on microbiome composition, accounting for 10% of community variation.[79] Of the medications reported in this study, the serotonin–norepinephrine reuptake inhibitor, venlafaxine, and the benzodiazepine, clonazepam, were the psychiatric medications included in the analysis. A thorough investigation of the effects of antidepressants on the gut microbiota has not been conducted in humans and it remains an unanswered question whether the bacteriocidal/bacteriostatic actions of psychotropic medication impact their efficacy or side effects.

SUMMARY AND PERSPECTIVES

Depression is a common, complex, heterogeneous disorder that encompasses the intricate interplay of biological and environmental factors. Converging data show that a complex network of lifelong microbial signaling pathways from gut to brain mediates many of the domains dysregulated in depression. Altered gut microbiota profiles have been demonstrated in depression. Moreover, FMT studies using GF and microbiota-depleted rodents suggest that the gut microbiota plays a physiological role. It remains an exciting frontier in psychiatric research to ascertain whether the gut microbiota and its metabolic output will serve as useful biosignatures to advance personalized precision treatment or preventive strategies in psychiatry. Furthermore, detailed investigation of the interaction among the gut microbiota, mood-regulating drugs, and nutrition in neuropsychiatric disorders is a promising avenue of clinical importance. We eagerly await prospective, rigorous, interventional clinical studies, using therapeutic modulation of the gut microbiota or its metabolites by psychobiotic strategies (probiotics, prebiotics, diet), with central markers of brain function.

REFERENCES

1. Dinan TG, Cryan JF. Melancholic microbes: a link between gut microbiota and depression? Neurogastroenterol Motil 2013;25(9):713–9.

2. Kelly JR, Minuto C, Cryan JF, et al. Cross talk: the microbiota and neurodevelopmental disorders. Front Neurosci 2017;11:490.

3. Erny D, Hrabe de Angelis AL, Jaitin D, et al. Host microbiota constantly control maturation and function of microglia in the CNS. Nat Neurosci 2015;18(7):965–77.

4. Sudo N, Chida Y, Aiba Y, et al. Postnatal microbial colonization programs the hypothalamic-pituitary-adrenal system for stress response in mice. J Physiol 2004;558(Pt 1):263–75.

5. O'Mahony SM, Clarke G, Borre YE, et al. Serotonin, tryptophan metabolism and the brain-gut-microbiome axis. Behav Brain Res 2015;277:32–48.

6. Stilling RM, van de Wouw M, Clarke G, et al. The neuropharmacology of butyrate: the bread and butter of the microbiota-gut-brain axis? Neurochem Int 2016;99: 110–32.

7. Bravo JA, Forsythe P, Chew MV, et al. Ingestion of *Lactobacillus* strain regulates emotional behavior and central GABA receptor expression in a mouse via the vagus nerve. Proc Natl Acad Sci U S A 2011;108(38):16050–5.

8. Arentsen T, Qian Y, Gkotzis S, et al. The bacterial peptidoglycan-sensing molecule Pglyrp2 modulates brain development and behavior. Mol Psychiatry 2017; 22(2):257–66.

9. WHO. Depression and other common mental disorders: global health estimates. Geneva (Switzerland). Licence: CC BY-NC-SA 3.0 IGO.

10. Kelly JR, Clarke G, Cryan JF, et al. Dimensional thinking in psychiatry in the era of the Research Domain Criteria (RDoC). Irish J Psychol Med 2018;35(2):89–94.

11. Bailey MT, Dowd SE, Galley JD, et al. Exposure to a social stressor alters the structure of the intestinal microbiota: implications for stressor-induced immunomodulation. Brain, Behav Immun 2011;25(3):397–407.

12. Vodička M, Ergang P, Hrnčíř T, et al. Microbiota affects the expression of genes involved in HPA axis regulation and local metabolism of glucocorticoids in chronic psychosocial stress. Brain Behav Immun 2018;73:615–24.

13. O'Mahony SM, Clarke G, Dinan TG, et al. Early-life adversity and brain development: is the microbiome a missing piece of the puzzle? Neuroscience 2017;342: 37–54.

14. De Palma G, Blennerhassett P, Lu J, et al. Microbiota and host determinants of behavioural phenotype in maternally separated mice. Nat Commun 2015;6:7735.

15. McVey Neufeld K-A, O'Mahony SM, Hoban AE, et al. Neurobehavioural effects of Lactobacillus rhamnosus GG alone and in combination with prebiotics polydextrose and galactooligosaccharide in male rats exposed to early-life stress. Nutr Neurosci 2019;22(6):425–34.

16. Golubeva AV, Crampton S, Desbonnet L, et al. Prenatal stress-induced alterations in major physiological systems correlate with gut microbiota composition in adulthood. Psychoneuroendocrinology 2015;60:58–74.

17. Jasarevic E, Howerton CL, Howard CD, et al. Alterations in the vaginal microbiome by maternal stress are associated with metabolic reprogramming of the offspring gut and brain. Endocrinol 2015;156:3265–76.

18. Jašarević E, Howard CD, Morrison K, et al. The maternal vaginal microbiome partially mediates the effects of prenatal stress on offspring gut and hypothalamus. Nat Neurosci 2018;21(8):1061–71.

19. Zijlmans MAC, Korpela K, Riksen-Walraven JM, et al. Maternal prenatal stress is associated with the infant intestinal microbiota. Psychoneuroendocrinology 2015; 53:233–45.

20. Lowry CA, Smith DG, Siebler PH, et al. The microbiota, immunoregulation, and mental health: implications for public health. Curr Environ Health Rep 2016; 3(3):270–86.

21. Dantzer R, Cohen S, Russo SJ, et al. Resilience and immunity. Brain Behav Immun 2018;74:28–42.

22. Reber SO, Siebler PH, Donner NC, et al. Immunization with a heat-killed preparation of the environmental bacterium Mycobacterium vaccae promotes stress resilience in mice. Proc Natl Acad Sci 2016;113(22):E3130–9.

23. Frank MG, Fonken LK, Dolzani SD, et al. Immunization with Mycobacterium vaccae induces an anti-inflammatory milieu in the CNS: attenuation of stress-induced microglial priming, alarmins and anxiety-like behavior. Brain Behav Immun 2018; 73:352–63.

24. Fox JH, Hassell JE, Siebler PH, et al. Preimmunization with a heat-killed preparation of Mycobacterium vaccae enhances fear extinction in the fear-potentiated startle paradigm. Brain Behav Immun 2017;66:70–84.

25. Siebler PH, Heinze JD, Kienzle DM, et al. Acute administration of the nonpathogenic, saprophytic bacterium, Mycobacterium vaccae, induces activation of

serotonergic neurons in the dorsal raphe nucleus and antidepressant-like behavior in association with mild hypothermia. Cell Mol Neurobiol 2018;38(1): 289–304.

26. Bollinger JL, Bergeon Burns CM, Wellman CL. Differential effects of stress on microglial cell activation in male and female medial prefrontal cortex. Brain Behav Immun 2016;52:88–97.

27. Codagnone MG, Spichak S, O'Mahony SM, et al. Programming bugs: microbiota and the developmental origins of brain health and disease. Biol Psychiatry 2019; 85(2):150–63.

28. Clarke G, Grenham S, Scully P, et al. The microbiome-gut-brain axis during early life regulates the hippocampal serotonergic system in a sex-dependent manner. Mol Psychiatry 2013;18(6):666–73.

29. Desbonnet L, Garrett L, Clarke G, et al. The probiotic *Bifidobacteria infantis*: an assessment of potential antidepressant properties in the rat. J Psychiatr Res 2008;43(2):164–74.

30. Reigstad CS, Salmonson CE, Rainey JF 3rd, et al. Gut microbes promote colonic serotonin production through an effect of short-chain fatty acids on enterochromaffin cells. Faseb J 2015;29(4):1395–403.

31. Yano JM, Yu K, Donaldson GP, et al. Indigenous bacteria from the gut microbiota regulate host serotonin biosynthesis. Cell 2015;161(2):264–76.

32. Schwarcz R, Stone TW. The kynurenine pathway and the brain: challenges, controversies and promises. Neuropharmacology 2017;112(Pt B):237–47.

33. Marin IA, Goertz JE, Ren T, et al. Microbiota alteration is associated with the development of stress-induced despair behavior. Scientific Rep 2017;7:43859.

34. Frost G, Sleeth ML, Sahuri-Arisoylu M, et al. The short-chain fatty acid acetate reduces appetite via a central homeostatic mechanism. Nat Commun 2014;5:3611.

35. Braniste V, Al-Asmakh M, Kowal C, et al. The gut microbiota influences blood-brain barrier permeability in mice. Sci Transl Med 2014;6(263):263ra158.

36. Frohlich EE, Farzi A, Mayerhofer R, et al. Cognitive impairment by antibiotic-induced gut dysbiosis: analysis of gut microbiota-brain communication. Brain Behav Immun 2016;56:140–55.

37. Schroeder FA, Lin CL, Crusio WE, et al. Antidepressant-like effects of the histone deacetylase inhibitor, sodium butyrate, in the mouse. Biol Psychiatry 2007;62(1): 55–64.

38. Wei Y, Melas PA, Wegener G, et al. Antidepressant-like effect of sodium butyrate is associated with an increase in TET1 and in 5-hydroxymethylation levels in the Bdnf gene. Int J Neuropsychopharmacol 2015;18(2) [pii:pyu032].

39. Gundersen BB, Blendy JA. Effects of the histone deacetylase inhibitor sodium butyrate in models of depression and anxiety. Neuropharmacology 2009;57(1): 67–74.

40. Gagliano H, Delgado-Morales R, Sanz-Garcia A, et al. High doses of the histone deacetylase inhibitor sodium butyrate trigger a stress-like response. Neuropharmacology 2014;79:75–82.

41. van de Wouw M, Boehme M, Lyte JM, et al. Short-chain fatty acids: microbial metabolites that alleviate stress-induced brain-gut axis alterations. J Physiol 2018; 596(20):4923–44.

42. Cowan CSM, Hoban AE, Ventura-Silva AP, et al. Gutsy moves: the amygdala as a critical node in microbiota to brain signaling. BioEssays 2018;40(1):1700172.

43. Luczynski P, Whelan SO, O'Sullivan C, et al. Adult microbiota-deficient mice have distinct dendritic morphological changes: differential effects in the amygdala and hippocampus. Eur J Neurosci 2016;44(9):2654–66.

44. Stilling RM, Ryan FJ, Hoban AE, et al. Microbes & neurodevelopment–Absence of microbiota during early life increases activity-related transcriptional pathways in the amygdala. Brain Behav Immun 2015;50:209–20.

45. Stilling RM, Moloney GM, Ryan FJ, et al. Social interaction-induced activation of RNA splicing in the amygdala of microbiome-deficient mice. Elife 2018;7 [pii: e33070].

46. Hoban AE, Stilling RM, Moloney G, et al. The microbiome regulates amygdala-dependent fear recall. Mol Psychiatry 2018;23(5):1134–44.

47. Hoban AE, Stilling RM, M Moloney G, et al. Microbial regulation of microRNA expression in the amygdala and prefrontal cortex. Microbiome 2017;5(1):102.

48. Hemmings SMJ, Malan-Muller S, van den Heuvel LL, et al. The microbiome in posttraumatic stress disorder and trauma-exposed controls: an exploratory study. Psychosom Med 2017;79(8):936–46.

49. Bach DR, Tzovara A, Vunder J. Blocking human fear memory with the matrix metalloproteinase inhibitor doxycycline. Mol Psychiatry 2018;23(7):1584–9.

50. Zheng P, Zeng B, Zhou C, et al. Gut microbiome remodeling induces depressive-like behaviors through a pathway mediated by the host's metabolism. Mol Psychiatry 2016;21(6):786–96.

51. Kelly JR, Borre Y, Brien C O', et al. Transferring the blues: depression-associated gut microbiota induces neurobehavioural changes in the rat. J Psychiatr Res 2016;82:109–18.

52. Yu M, Jia H, Zhou C, et al. Variations in gut microbiota and fecal metabolic phenotype associated with depression by 16S rRNA gene sequencing and LC/MS-based metabolomics. J Pharm Biomed Anal 2017;138:231–9.

53. Evans SJ, Bassis CM, Hein R, et al. The gut microbiome composition associates with bipolar disorder and illness severity. J Psychiatr Res 2017;87:23–9.

54. Jiang H, Ling Z, Zhang Y, et al. Altered fecal microbiota composition in patients with major depressive disorder. Brain Behav Immun 2015;48:186–94.

55. Liu Y, Zhang L, Wang X, et al. Similar fecal microbiota signatures in patients with diarrhea-predominant irritable bowel syndrome and patients with depression. Clin Gastroenterol Hepatol 2016;14(11):1602–11.e5.

56. De Palma G, Lynch MD. Transplantation of fecal microbiota from patients with irritable bowel syndrome alters gut function and behavior in recipient mice. Sci Transl Med 2017;9(379) [pii: eaaf6397].

57. Dinan TG, Stanton C, Cryan JF. Psychobiotics: a novel class of psychotropic. Biol Psychiatry 2013;74(10):720–6.

58. Sarkar A, Lehto SM, Harty S, et al. Psychobiotics and the manipulation of bacteria–gut–brain signals. Trends Neurosciences 2016;39(11):763–81.

59. Kelly JR, Clarke G, Cryan JF, et al. Brain-gut-microbiota axis: challenges for translation in psychiatry. Ann Epidemiol 2016;26(5):366–72.

60. Kelly JR, Allen AP, Temko A, et al. Lost in translation? The potential psychobiotic Lactobacillus rhamnosus (JB-1) fails to modulate stress or cognitive performance in healthy male subjects. Brain Behav Immun 2017;61:50–9.

61. Kelly JR, Kennedy PJ, Cryan JF, et al. Breaking down the barriers: the gut microbiome, intestinal permeability and stress-related psychiatric disorders. Front Cell Neurosci 2015;9:392.

62. Zmora N, Zilberman-Schapira G, Suez J, et al. Personalized gut mucosal colonization resistance to empiric probiotics is associated with unique host and microbiome features. Cell 2018;174(6):1388–405.e21.

63. Akkasheh G, Kashani-Poor Z, Tajabadi-Ebrahimi M, et al. Clinical and metabolic response to probiotic administration in patients with major depressive disorder: a randomized, double-blind, placebo-controlled trial. Nutrition 2016;32(3):315–20.

64. Romijn AR, Rucklidge JJ, Kuijer RG, et al. A double-blind, randomized, placebo-controlled trial of Lactobacillus helveticus and Bifidobacterium longum for the symptoms of depression. Aust N Z J Psychiatry 2017;51(8):810–21.

65. Dickerson F, Adamos M, Katsafanas E, et al. Adjunctive probiotic microorganisms to prevent rehospitalization in patients with acute mania: a randomized controlled trial. Bipolar Disord 2018;20(7):614–21.

66. Pinto-Sanchez MI, Hall GB, Ghajar K, et al. Probiotic Bifidobacterium longum NCC3001 reduces depression scores and alters brain activity: a pilot study in patients with irritable bowel syndrome. Gastroenterology 2017;153(2):448–59.e8.

67. Labus JS, Hollister EB, Jacobs J, et al. Differences in gut microbial composition correlate with regional brain volumes in irritable bowel syndrome. Microbiome 2017;5(1):49.

68. Patterson E, RM OD, Murphy EF, et al. Impact of dietary fatty acids on metabolic activity and host intestinal microbiota composition in C57BL/6J mice. Br J Nutr 2014;111(11):1905–17.

69. Robertson RC, Seira Oriach C, Murphy K, et al. Omega-3 polyunsaturated fatty acids critically regulate behaviour and gut microbiota development in adolescence and adulthood. Brain Behav Immun 2017;59:21–37.

70. Weiser MJ, Wynalda K, Salem N Jr, et al. Dietary DHA during development affects depression-like behaviors and biomarkers that emerge after puberty in adolescent rats. J lipid Res 2015;56(1):151–66.

71. Robertson RC, Seira Oriach C, Murphy K, et al. Deficiency of essential dietary n-3 PUFA disrupts the caecal microbiome and metabolome in mice. Br J Nutr 2017; 118(11):959–70.

72. Jacka FN. Nutritional psychiatry: where to next? EBioMedicine 2017;17:24–9.

73. Opie RS, Itsiopoulos C, Parletta N, et al. Dietary recommendations for the prevention of depression. Nutr Neurosci 2017;20(3):161–71.

74. De Filippis F, Pellegrini N, Vannini L, et al. High-level adherence to a Mediterranean diet beneficially impacts the gut microbiota and associated metabolome. Gut 2016;65(11):1812–21.

75. Lassale C, Batty GD, Baghdadli A, et al. Healthy dietary indices and risk of depressive outcomes: a systematic review and meta-analysis of observational studies. Mol Psychiatry 2018. [Epub ahead of print].

76. Oddy WH, Allen KL, Trapp GSA, et al. Dietary patterns, body mass index and inflammation: pathways to depression and mental health problems in adolescents. Brain Behav Immun 2018;69:428–39.

77. Khambadkone SG, Cordner ZA, Dickerson F, et al. Nitrated meat products are associated with mania in humans and altered behavior and brain gene expression in rats. 2018.

78. Cussotto S, Strain CR, Fouhy F, et al. Differential effects of psychotropic drugs on microbiome composition and gastrointestinal function. Psychopharmacology (Berl) 2018. [Epub ahead of print].

79. Falony G, Joossens M, Vieira-Silva S, et al. Population-level analysis of gut microbiome variation. Science 2016;352(6285):560–4.

80. Naseribafrouei A, Hestad K, Avershina E, et al. Correlation between the human fecal microbiota and depression. Neurogastroenterol Motil 2014;26(8):1155–62.

The Role of the Gut-Brain Axis in Attention-Deficit/ Hyperactivity Disorder

Sarita A. Dam, MSc[a],*, Jeanette C. Mostert, PhD[b],
Joanna W. Szopinska-Tokov, MSc[c], Mirjam Bloemendaal, PhD[c],
Maria Amato, MSc[b], Alejandro Arias-Vasquez, PhD[b,c]

KEYWORDS

- Gut-brain axis • Endocrine communication • Immunology • Metabolites
- Nerval communication • Biomarkers • ADHD • Genetics

KEY POINTS

- Attention-deficit/hyperactivity disorder (ADHD) is a heterogeneous genetic neurodevelopmental disorder, currently mainly treated with medication. Dietary interventions are promising nonpharmacologic interventions for ADHD.
- The gut-brain axis is a bidirectional communication mechanism between the gut and the brain that includes nerval (ie, the vagus nerve), endocrine, and immunologic pathways.
- Vagal nerve activity is a potential pathophysiologic mechanism for ADHD, which is partially driven by the signals triggered by the commensal bacteria (microbiota) via cells in gut epithelium.
- The gut microbiota could play an important role in ADHD by affecting the synthesis and metabolism of dopamine, serotonin, noradrenalin, gamma-aminobutyric acid, and other neurotransmitters and their precursors.

Continued

Disclosure Statement: None of the authors have actual or potential conflict of interest in relation to this publication.

Funding: The research leading to these results received funding from the European Community's Horizon 2020 research and innovation programme under the Marie Sklodowska-Curie grant agreement no. 643051 (MiND) and under grant agreement no. 728018 (Eat2BeNICE), and the Netherlands Organisation for Scientific Research (NWO) Food Cognition and Behavior Program in relation to the B3: Brain, Bacteria & Behavior project (grant agreement number 057–14–005) and Radboudumc Junior researcher round 2018 Donders Centre for Medical Neuroscience(DCMN).

[a] Department of Cognitive Neuroscience, Donders Institute for Brain, Cognition and Behaviour, Radboud University Medical Center, Kapittelweg 29, 6525 EN, Nijmegen, The Netherlands; [b] Department of Human Genetics, Donders Institute for Brain, Cognition and Behaviour, Radboud University Medical Center, Geert Grooteplein Zuid 10, 6525 GA, Nijmegen, The Netherlands; [c] Department of Psychiatry, Donders Institute for Brain, Cognition and Behaviour, Radboud University Medical Center, Geert Grooteplein Zuid 10, 6525 GA, Nijmegen, The Netherlands
* Corresponding author.
E-mail address: Sarita.Dam@radboudumc.nl

Continued

- Immunologic homeostasis, regulated by host genetics and (partially) educated by the gut microbiota, relates to ADHD prevalence, clinical symptoms, and cognitive functioning in ADHD.

INTRODUCTION

For a long time, the brain was considered as the only important organ in understanding the biology of neuropsychiatric disorders. Recently, this focus has shifted to include the gut.[1] The gut-brain axis (GBA) is a continuous, bidirectional communication system between the enteric nervous system (ENS) and the cognitive and emotional centers of the brain.[2] A key modifier of the GBA is the gut microbiota, which refers to the microorganisms that colonize the human gastrointestinal tract after birth.[3] The gut microorganisms and their genes (collectively called the gut microbiome) are transferred from mother to baby at birth and continue to mature during the first years of life,[4] before reaching a certain stability. Throughout the lifespan, this stability is susceptible to a variety of factors (eg, host genetics, diet, stress, medication, and illness).[3]

With new DNA sequencing techniques, we are now able to readily investigate the composition of the microbiome, that is, the genome of the gut microbiota. These techniques provide new avenues to investigate the role that the gut plays in behavior and mental health.[5] In this review, the authors focus on attention-deficit/hyperactivity disorder (ADHD). This neurodevelopmental disorder is influenced by both genetic and environmental factors that interact with the GBA. The gut microbiome is therefore a likely candidate for identifying (not yet available) ADHD biomarkers. The authors first provide a brief overview of the clinical and biological picture of ADHD and then discuss various routes of communication from the gut to the brain that play a role in the development and treatment of ADHD.

THE CLINICAL PICTURE OF ATTENTION-DEFICIT/HYPERACTIVITY DISORDER

ADHD is a clinically heterogeneous neurodevelopmental disorder that starts in childhood and can persist into adulthood.[6] The world-wide prevalence of ADHD is estimated to be around 5% in children[7] and 2.5% in adults.[8] In children, the disorder is characterized by excessive, persistent, and age-inappropriate symptoms of inattention, hyperactivity, and/or impulsivity that interfere with daily functioning and development (see **Box 1** for the DSM-5 symptom list).[6] During adolescence, hyperactive and impulsive symptoms decline in most individuals, whereas inattentive symptoms remain or even increase toward adulthood.[9]

In children, ADHD is 2 to 3 times more prevalent in boys than in girls,[10] while in adults prevalence is (almost) equal between genders.[11] Genetic and neuroendocrine factors are likely factors to contribute to sex differences in childhood ADHD diagnosis,[12] but an overdiagnosis of boys and underdiagnosis of girls should not be excluded. In adulthood, sex differences are still apparent in the prevalence and type of comorbid disorders.[11,13]

The most frequent comorbidities presenting with ADHD include autism spectrum disorders,[14] tics,[15] learning disorders,[16] rule-breaking behaviors (including oppositional defiant or conduct disorders[17,18]), substance use disorders,[19] mood and anxiety

---

Box 1
DSM-5 diagnostic criteria for attention-deficit/hyperactivity disorder

A. A persistent pattern of inattention and/or hyperactivity-impulsivity that interferes with functioning or development, as characterized by (1) and/or (2):

1. Inattention: 6 (or more) of the following symptoms of inattention have persisted for at least 6 months to a degree that is inconsistent with developmental level and that negatively affects directly on social and academic/occupational activities[a]:

   i. Often fails to give close attention to details or makes careless mistakes in schoolwork, at work, or during other activities
   ii. Often has difficulty sustaining attention in tasks or play activities
   iii. Often does not seem to listen when spoken to directly
   iv. Often does not follow through on instructions and fails to finish school work, chores, or duties in the workplace
   v. Often has difficulty organizing tasks and activities
   vi. Often avoids, dislikes, or is reluctant to engage in tasks that require sustained mental effort
   vii. Often loses things necessary for tasks or activities
   viii. Is often easily distracted by extraneous stimuli
   ix. Is often forgetful in daily activities

2. Hyperactivity and impulsivity: 6 (or more) of the following symptoms of hyperactivity-impulsivity have persisted for at least 6 months to a degree that is inconsistent with developmental level and that negatively affects directly on social and academic/occupational activities[a]:

   i. Often fidgets with or taps hands or feet or squirms in seat
   ii. Often leaves seat in classroom or in other situations in which remaining seated is expected
   iii. Often runs about or climbs excessively in situations in which it is inappropriate (in adolescents or adults, may be limited to subjective feelings of restless)
   iv. Often unable to play or engage in leisure activities quietly
   v. Is often "on the go," acting as if "driven by a motor"
   vi. Often talks excessively
   vii. Often blurts out an answer before a question has been completed
   viii. Often has difficulty awaiting his or her turn
   ix. Often interrupts or intrudes on others

B. Several hyperactive-impulsive or inattentive symptoms that caused impairment were present before age 12 years.

C. Several inattentive or hyperactive-impulsive symptoms are present in 2 or more settings (eg, at home, school, or work; with friends or relatives; in other activities).

D. There is clear evidence that the symptoms interfere with, or reduce the quality of, social, academic, or occupational functioning.

E. The symptoms do not occur exclusively during the course of schizophrenia or another psychotic disorder and are not better explained by another mental disorder (eg, mood disorder, anxiety disorder, dissociative disorder, personality disorder, substance intoxication, or withdrawal).

[a] For older adolescents and adults (aged 17 years and older), at least 5 symptoms are required.

---

disorders,[20] bipolar disorder, [21] and emotional liability.[22] Furthermore, somatic conditions such as obesity,[23] type-2 diabetes,[13] and autoimmune diseases, including Crohn disease,[24] are also more prevalent in individuals with ADHD compared with those without. Interestingly, population, family, and twin studies show significant genetic correlation between ADHD (and other psychiatric and neurodevelopmental disorders) with these somatic conditions, hence increasing the risk for the onset of multiple disorders.[25]

THE BIOLOGY OF ATTENTION-DEFICIT/HYPERACTIVITY DISORDER
Genetics

ADHD shows substantial heritability, which is estimated at ~76% through multiple twin studies.[26] The genetic architecture of ADHD is complex, with multiple different genetic variants contributing to the disorder,[27] both common and rare.[28]

Given the multifactorial, polygenic nature of ADHD, genetic research has mainly focused on common variants through hypothesis-driven candidate gene association studies and hypothesis-free genome-wide association studies (GWAS).[27,28] Candidate gene studies of ADHD have mainly focused on genes related to neurotransmission systems, such as the dopamine transporter (DAT1), dopamine receptors (DRD4 and 5), serotonin transporter (5HTT) and serotonin receptor (5HT1B), and neuronal development genes such as SNAP25.[29] However, because of the heterogeneous nature of ADHD and methodological differences between studies, findings have often been inconclusive and difficult to replicate.[29] Recently, a genome-wide association meta-analysis identified, for the first time, 12 significant genome-wide risk markers for ADHD through the combination of several very large cohorts.[30] Although the identified markers were mainly located in or near genes related to neurodevelopment, none of the pre-GWAS most-studied genetic "suspects" have been "rediscovered" (yet) via GWAS. Importantly, a significant proportion of these associated genetic variants are not unique to ADHD but correlate with other psychiatric (ie, depression) and somatic disorders (ie, obesity) and explain only a very small portion of the genetic risk for ADHD.[30]

Neurobiology

Pathways leading toward ADHD are hypothesized to be mediated by alterations in diverse brain networks.[25] A recent neuroimaging mega-analysis reported subtle but consistent reduction in volumes of subcortical brain regions and intracranial volume in ADHD compared with healthy controls.[31] How such alterations contribute to the disease phenotype is still poorly understood.

Brain networks implicated in ADHD (see[32–34] for details) are innervated by neurotransmitters that play an important role in ADHD (eg, noradrenalin, dopamine, gamma-aminobutyric acid [GABA], and serotonin).[35–37] Impaired function of these regions (**Fig. 1**), or the connectivity between them, is thought to underlie many of the ADHD symptoms, including poor inhibition of (motor) actions (resulting in hyperactivity and impulsivity), impaired sensitivity for reward and motivation, and problems with attention and working memory.[32,38,39]

ENVIRONMENTAL EFFECTS ON ATTENTION-DEFICIT/HYPERACTIVITY DISORDER

ADHD is a highly heritable disease. Nevertheless, relevant environmental factors have been associated with ADHD risk. Prenatal factors (maternal stress, smoking, and alcohol use during pregnancy), perinatal factors (stress, low birth weight, premature birth, breastfeeding), exposure to environmental toxins, and maltreatment have been robustly characterized with disease risk.[40–43] These environmental effects can contribute directly to ADHD risk (eg, maternal smoking/alcohol use during pregnancy) or indirectly by, for example, modifying gene functions through epigenetic changes, especially in genetically susceptible individuals.[41] Interactions between genes and environmental factors are known to play a substantial role in ADHD development, although a complete understanding of these factors and their interactions is still lacking.[44]

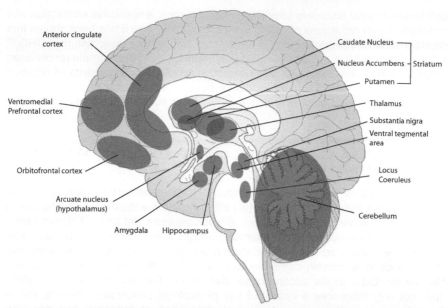

Fig. 1. Brain regions implicated in ADHD. Grey-shaded areas indicate brain regions that have been implicated in ADHD pathophysiology. Neurotransmitters are released from neurons that originate in the brainstem and midbrain (eg, locus coeruleus, substantia nigra, ventral tegmental area) and project to various subcortical (eg, amygdala, hippocampus, thalamus, caudate nucleus, putamen, nucleus accumbens) and cortical regions (eg, cerebellum, anterior cingulate cortex, ventromedial prefrontal cortex and orbitofrontal cortex).

TREATMENT OF ATTENTION-DEFICIT/HYPERACTIVITY DISORDER
Pharmacologic Treatments of Attention-Deficit/Hyperactivity Disorder

Current first-choice ADHD treatments are stimulants (methylphenidate and amphetamines), followed by nonstimulants (atomoxetine, guanfacine, and clonidine).[25,45,46] These treatments mainly target dopamine, noradrenalin, and serotonin neurotransmitter systems by blocking their reuptake transporters (dopamine in the case of methylphenidate and amphetamines, noradrenalin by atomoxetine), thereby increasing neurotransmitter availability in the synaptic cleft.[47] In many patients, pharmacologic treatment (usually given in combination with nonpharmacologic interventions) is effective in reducing ADHD symptoms.[45,48,49] However, not all patients respond well to medication (one study estimated efficacy of stimulant medication around 70%[50]) or may not tolerate adverse effects.[45,51]

Nonpharmacologic Interventions for Attention Deficit Hyperactivity Disorder

Nonpharmacologic treatments generally have smaller effect sizes compared with pharmacologic treatment, but may be very important for those patients who do not respond well to medication[52,53] or those who present with adverse effects. Interventions such as behavioral therapy, cognitive training, neurofeedback, mindfulness, or diet are currently used in the control and management of ADHD.[54–58] Recently, dietary interventions seem to be a promising avenue to significantly reduce disease symptomatology.[59–61] Food intake can affect brain development and function in all age groups, starting in utero, and influence cognitive processes, mood, and brain performance.[62] Several studies have also linked nutritional components to neurodevelopmental disorders specifically. For instance, a restrictive elimination diet is associated with reductions of ADHD symptoms,[52,63,64] and it has been shown that a Western-style diet in adolescents is associated with an increased risk for ADHD.[65] However, findings have not been consistently replicated in large sample randomized controlled trials,[66] and the effect sizes of active/protective components of nutrition have not been determined through evidence-based methods, nor are interindividual differences or the mechanisms underlying effects of such components completely understood.[67]

INTESTINAL BACTERIA AS A MECHANISTIC LINK BETWEEN DIET AND ATTENTION-DEFICIT/HYPERACTIVITY DISORDER

Diet might influence ADHD-related behavioral processes acting directly on the enteric nervous sytem or indirectly by (ie,) affecting the composition and functioning of the gut microbiome.[68] In the first case, the link between diet and ADHD symptomatology could be explained by, for example, allergic reactions to food: children with ADHD have an increased risk of developing allergies,[69,70] meaning that an abnormal immune reaction to certain components could affect the central nervous system (CNS) via the GBA. In the second case, diet affects the gut microbiome,[68] which in turn not only influences a variety of key physiologic processes (appetite, metabolism, immune system, processing, and absorption of nutrients) but has also been shown to influence brain chemistry and neural development through the GBA in several psychiatric diseases.[5] This is supported by animal studies showing that swapping microbes from one timid group of mice into the guts of mice who tended to take more risks, and vice versa, generated a complete personality shift: timid mice became outgoing, whereas outgoing mice became timid.[71] The authors' own work, performed by Tengeler and colleagues (Tengeler AC, Dam SA, Wiesmann M, et al. Gut microbiota from persons with attention-deficit/hyperactivity disorder affects brain structure and behavior in mice. submitted) (manuscript in preparation), shows that germ-free (GF) mice (mice reared in the absence of microbial colonization) colonized with microbiota from adult patients with ADHD were more anxious and showed altered brain structure and connectivity compared with mice colonized with healthy control microbiome. Similar research on ADHD in humans is still scarce; fecal transplant is not a real treatment option for neurodevelopmental disorders (NDDs), but a longitudinal randomized control study showed that children treated with a perinatal probiotic intervention were less likely to be diagnosed with ADHD at a later age.[72] In addition, the authors' own work found microbiome alterations in ADHD and microbiome-produced monoamine precursors to be related to decreased ventral striatal functional MRI responses during reward anticipation.[73] To the authors' knowledge, this latter study is the only one to date linking microbiome alterations in ADHD with alteration in brain activity. Although the specific mechanism through which the microbiome is able to mediate this effect has not been investigated, there is evidence for the existence of various routes through which the microbiome can affect behavior and brain homeostasis.

In the next part of this review, the authors discuss 3 of these routes via which the microbiota can mediate the brain and behavior and present the current knowledge on 3 key mechanisms underlying the complex communication between microbiome, gut, and brain in relation to ADHD: (1) the link between gut and brain via the vagus nerve [VN],[74] (2) the interaction between the microbiome with the host's (epi)genome and metabolome through the synthesis of neurotransmittors and metabolites,[3] and (3) interaction with the host's immunologic system[75] (Fig. 2).

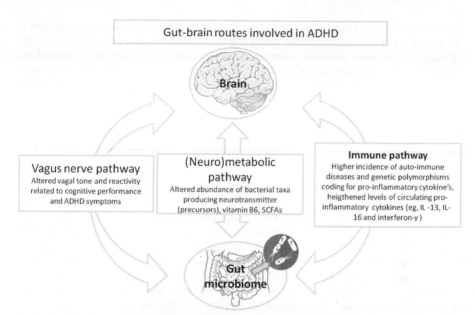

Fig. 2. Gut-brain routes implicated in ADHD. Depicted are 3 routes and the main mechanisms via which the gut microbiota can influence the brain and behavior. From left to right: communication via the vagus nerve, the (neuro)metabolic pathway, and the immune pathway. Each of these routes is discussed in this review in more detail.

Pathway 1: the Role of the Vagus Nerve in Gut-Brain Axis

The VN is the 10th cranial nerve and the main component of the parasympathetic nervous system, which is involved in key functions (eg, control of mood, immune response, appetite and digestion via intestinal permeability and enteric reflex, and heart rate) and influences the hypothalamic-pituitary-adrenal axis (HPA axis; involved in stress regulation).[76–80] The VN consists of afferent (80%–90%) and efferent 10%-20% fibers[81] that interact with the (microbiota-rich) colonic mucosa layer[74] via mechanoreceptors, chemoreceptors, and tension receptors.[76,80,82,83] The fibers that conduct sensory impulses from the gut to the CNS (afferent fibers) can sense only indirect microbiota signals, through the diffusion of bacterial compounds or metabolites, or thanks to other cells (ie, enteroendocrine cells) located in the epithelium.[74,80,83] From these cells information is passed on to the VN by releasing the neurotransmitter glutamate, which sends it to the nucleus tractus solitarii (NTS), found in the brainstem, within milliseconds.[84,85] This nucleus then sends this sensory information to several cortical and subcortical regions of the CNS (eg, the rostral ventrolateral medulla, the amygdala, the hippocampus, the ventral prefrontal cortex, the arcuate nucleus, and the thalamus).[78,83,86] Importantly, monoamine nuclei in the brainstem, the locus coeruleus (major source of noradrenalin projections throughout the CNS), and the raphe nuclei (a diffusely serotonergic projecting system that innervates virtually all areas of the CNS) receive direct and/or indirect projections from the NTS.[87–89]

Evidence supporting the role of the VN as a player in the GBA comes from several studies. Cussotto and colleagues[78] and Klarer and colleagues,[90] demonstrated that inactivation of specific vagal afferents decreased social deficits in mice and decreased innate anxiety and learned fear in rats—emotions that are both subjected to visceral modulation through abdominal vagal afferents. Recently, Nishigaki and colleagues[91] showed that treating young mice with monosodium glutamate (a popular ingredient in processed foods to enhance flavor) leads to a reduced emotional behavior later in life, especially aggression, and that vagotomy at the subdiaphragmatic level blocked the effect of the stimulant on this behavior.[92] They suggested that the VN action is mediated at least in part by gut-brain interaction, as it is very likely that monosodium glutamate ingestion changed the pattern of microbiota, which influenced the activity of the VN.[83,91,93]

THE ROLE OF THE VAGUS NERVE IN ATTENTION-DEFICIT/HYPERACTIVITY DISORDER

It is not yet clear if VN dysregulation is directly involved in the pathophysiology of ADHD. However, several deficits observed in ADHD can (also) be modulated by the VN. Firstly, it has been shown that a gut-to-brain neural circuit establishes vagal neurons as an essential component of the reward neuronal pathway, which uses dopamine signaling and is altered in patients with ADHD.[73,85] Several studies have reported altered activity and/or reactivity of the parasympathetic nervous system in ADHD, but findings are inconsistent.[94] Rash and Aguirre-Camacho[95] performed a systematic review on vagal reactivity and has previously reported tentative evidence that children with unmedicated ADHD display lower levels of vagal tone. In addition, children with ADHD showed an augmented pattern of vagal reactivity (compared with controls), when performing tasks involving self-regulation and regulation of emotions.[92] Similarly, a moderated vagal reactivity was associated with short-term memory performance and ADHD diagnosis (independently of comorbidity) in a sample of children with ADHD and healthy controls.[96] Koenig and colleagues[96] provided evidence for alterations of long-term and nocturnal vagal activity in children with ADHD, which might arise from circadian rhythm sleep disorders. More recently, Sandgren and Bummer[97], however, reported that VN activity is elevated in patients with ADHD. They provide clinical evidence indicating that peripheral arousal and amplification of incoming sensory information affect attention and distractibility in patients with ADHD at a lower processing level (ie, at the locus coeruleus).[98,99] Aston-Jones and colleagues[100,101] also observed that ADHD may result, at least in part, from an overly tonic locus coeruleus mode. As the tonic locus coeruleus mode facilitates interactions with many stimuli rather than focusing on only a subset, this could produce an inability to focus attention. Finally, previous work showed a role of the VN in learning and memory functioning[102–104] in which a physiologic role for vagal sensory signaling from the gut was established.[105] However, the role of VN on learning and memory is inconclusive and it seems that it depends on the task conditions, indicating that the relative contribution of vagal afferent signaling is most evident in conditions that require subjects to adapt their cognitive strategies to face new and unexpected changes in the environment,[106] something that also seems affected in patients with ADHD.

Pathway 2: the Role of (Neuro)metabolites in the Gut-Brain Axis and Attention Deficit Hyperactivity Disorder

In this section, the authors describe the neurotransmitters that are targeted by ADHD medication (dopamine, serotonin, noradrenalin, or GABA), their precursors, and other metabolites as factors that are involved in ADHD pathogenesis and how these factors are linked to the GBA through the gut microbiota as a main player. It is important to note that there are other (not yet identified) potential factors involved in the GBA homeostasis with downstream effects on NDDs. At this point, their roles are unclear, unknown, or less relevant for ADHD, so they are not included in this review.

DOPAMINE, NORADRENALIN, SEROTONIN, AND GAMMA-AMINOBUTYRIC ACID
Dopamine and Noradrenalin

Dopamine and noradrenalin are involved in ADHD pathophysiology and play essential roles in behavioral, cognitive, and affective functions.[107,108] Dopamine, noradrenalin, and their precursors can be produced by the gut microbiota.[109,110] Asano and colleagues[111] showed that the levels of both dopamine and noradrenalin are significantly decreased in germ-free (GF) mice. More importantly, this could be reversed (significant increased levels in the gut) with a fecal transplant into these mice. Moreover, the gut microbiota seems to be involved in the mRNA expression of the dopamine D1 receptor, which was significantly higher in the hippocampus in GF mice and showed a higher turnover rate in the striatum.[112] This shows that the gut-produced dopamine and noradrenalin can have brain level effects. In a study using patients with ADHD, Aarts and colleagues[73] found that the bacterial genus *Bifidobacterium* was increased in persons with ADHD compared with controls and that was linked with an enzyme involved in the phenylalanine synthesis, a precursor of dopamine.

Serotonin

Serotonin has been found in numerous (pre)clinical studies to play an important factor in ADHD pathogenesis.[37,113–115] The role of serotonin in the GBA is especially worth investigating, as around 90% of the body serotonin is made in the gut mainly by enterochromaffin cells, and gut microbiota promote this biosynthesis by sending signals to them[116,117] or producing serotonin on their own (**Box 2**[118]). Considerable evidence indicates that serotonin released from enterochromaffin cells can send signals to the CNS.[116,119,120] However, intestinal serotonin has yet to be linked directly to brain function in ADHD. Mechanistically, gut microbiota can change the peripheral availability of tryptophan.[121] Tryptophan can subsequently cross the blood-brain barrier (BBB) affecting serotonin synthesis in CNS.[122,123] A clinical study showed that ADHD had lower circulating serotonin concentration, which was also observed in GF mice,[124] and that oral administration of tryptophan alleviates ADHD symptoms.[37]

Box 2
Serotonin-producing bacterial strains
Bacterial strain
Lactococcus lactis subsp. cremoris (MG 1363)
L. lactis subsp. lactis (IL1403)
Lactobacillus plantarum (FI8595)
Streptococcus thermophilus (NCFB2392)
Escherichia coli K-12
Morganella morganii (NCIMB, 10466)
Klebsiella pneumoniae (NCIMB, 673)
Hafnia alvei (NCIMB, 11999)
From O'Mahony SM, Clarke G, Borre YE, Dinan TG, Cryan JF. Serotonin, tryptophan metabolism and the brain-gut-microbiome axis. Behav Brain Res 2015;277:32-48; with permission.

Gamma-Aminobutyric Acid

(Pre)clinical studies showed GABA as another important key factor that may contribute to the pathology of ADHD.[36,125–127] In general, gut microbiota influences the availability of GABA to the CNS through secretion and absorption of this neurotransmitter.[120,128] Specifically, several commensal organisms have been reported to produce GABA, including members of the Bifidobacterium, Lactobacillus, and Escherichia coli.[129–131] Of those known, Lactobacillus rhamnosus JB-1 is most often cited, as it was found that its introduction into mice reduced depressive- and anxiety-like behavior in a vagus-dependent manner, with accompanying changes in cerebral GABAergic activity.[93] A study administering probiotics to persons with ADHD showed that early intervention with Lactobacillus may reduce the risk of ADHD development later in childhood,[72] by increasing the level of GABA.[132] Furthermore, taxonomical microbiome studies showed increased Bifidobacterium in adults with ADHD,[73] but it is not clear if those GABA-producing bacteria drove this result. Recently, it was showed that Bacteroides spp. produce large quantities of GABA[133] and the relative abundance of the certain species belonging to this genus were increased in ADHD.[73] Parabacteroides and Prevotella seem to be GABA-producing bacteria[134] and were found to be decreased in ADHD.[135] This shows the relevance of studying the gut microbiome in relation to GABA involvement in ADHD pathogenesis.

Other Relevant Bacterial Metabolic Factors for Attention Deficit Hyperactivity Disorder

In addition to producing neurotransmitters and their precursors, gut microbiota produces vitamins.[136] One of these is vitamin B6,[137] a coenzyme involved in neurotransmitter metabolism and synthesis.[138] Impaired activity of B6-dependent enzymes have been found in patients with ADHD.[139] Moreover, the serum concentration of vitamin B6 was found to be lower in ADHD.[140,141] Mousain-Bosc and colleagues[142] showed that ingestion of vitamin B6 with magnesium improved ADHD symptoms in children, which raises the question if patients with ADHD lack B6-producing bacteria.[97]

Other important bacterial metabolites are the short-chain fatty acids (SCFAs), major products of bacterial fermentation from dietary fiber, which have various effects on the host brain and behavior.[143] For instance, SCFAs increase the rate-limiting enzymes in dopamine and noradrenalin synthesis (via tyrosine hydroxylase expression) and serotonin synthesis (via tryptophan hydroxylase expression) and lower GABA levels.[144] This suggests that SCFAs are involved in modulating neurotransmission and unsurprisingly, are associated with deficits in cognition and sociability.[145] SCFAs are also capable of influencing BBB permeability, although, the mechanism is still unknown.[146] BBB is a highly selective semipermeable interface that separates the brain interior from the peripheral blood and controls the transport of molecules in and out of the brain.[147]

Disruption of this BBB has been suggested as an underlying mechanism in psychiatric disorders, including ADHD.[147,148] In addition, gut microbiota are capable of changing BBB permeability, possibly by changing the expression of tight junction proteins occludin and claudin-5.[149]

Although not a metabolic product of the gut microbiota, the structural signatures of the bacterial wall can be recognized by the host immune systems. Peptidoglycan, a component of bacterial cell wall, can cross the BBB.[150] A seminal study by Arentsen and colleagues[150] showed that human immune system has receptors that detect peptidoglycan, and these receptors can be activated at the brain level, proving that bacterial signaling can go all the way to the brain and influence its development.

Pathway 3: the Role of the Immune System in the Gut-Brain Axis and Attention Deficit Hyperactivity Disorder

The host immune system rapidly responds to the infection coming from the gut microbiota in an antigen nonspecific manner through the activation of pattern recognition receptors. This starts the release of cytokines such as interferon alpha, interleukin 18 (IL-18), and IL-22 to promote epithelial antimicrobial responses such as the production of antimicrobial peptides.[151] Immune recognition of gut microbiota is shown to trigger multiple inflammatory disorders. For example, both mucosal and serum antibodies targeting gut commensal antigens are elevated in individuals with Crohn disease and those with ulcerative colitis.[152,153]

The mediating routes of the immune system in the GBA are currently being mapped. These routes include peripheral cytokines passing through the BBB centrally acting on toll-like receptors located on neuronal cells and microglia to produce more cytokines.[154,155] Neuroinflammation subsequently results in impaired barrier function both at the intestine and the brain, reduced synaptic pruning, neuronal damage through oxidative stress, and reduced neurotransmitter availability.[156–158] Gut immune functioning has indeed been implicated in a range of psychiatric, neurodegenerative, and neurodevelopmental diseases[159]; patients with immune-related disorders such as inflammatory bowel syndrome often have comorbid disorders such as anxiety and depression disorder.[160] Vice versa, in depressed patients, gut microbiota alterations and higher level of proinflammatory cytokines and antibodies co-occur.[161–163] For neurodevelopmental disorders, autism spectrum disorder is associated with immune dysregulations such as infection during pregnancy and early life.[5,164]

EPIDEMIOLOGIC STUDIES SHOW COMORBIDITY OF AUTOIMMUNE DISORDERS AND ATTENTION-DEFICIT/HYPERACTIVITY DISORDERS

Evidence is emerging that gut immune dysfunctions are part of the pathophysiology of ADHD.[148] An increased incidence for atopic diseases such as eczema, Crohn disease, allergic rhinitis, asthma, atopic dermatitis, and allergic conjunctivitis are observed in patients with ADHD[113,165,166] with prominent gender differences for increased versus reduced prevalence for Crohn disease in women versus men.[24] Also, the reverse is observed in larger samples: in patients with atopic diseases, symptom severity relates to increased ADHD prevalence, indicating shared genetic predisposition between atopic diseases and ADHD.[167,168]

GENETIC POLYMORPHISMS INVOLVED IN IMMUNE FUNCTIONING ARE LINKED TO ATTENTION-DEFICIT/HYPERACTIVITY DISORDER PATHOLOGY

The 4-repeat allele of the IL-1 receptor antagonist gene is associated with an increased risk for ADHD and the 2-repeat with a reduced risk.[169] Also, the IL-6 and tumor necrosis factor alpha (TNF-α) genes have been associated with child ADHD and cognitive measures for visuomotor coordination and attention, respectively.[170] Furthermore, the IL-16 gene was associated with the ADHD inattentive subtype and nuclear factor, IL-3 regulated with earlier onset of ADHD.[171,172] Smith and colleagues[173] showed that the IL-16 gene modulates the relation between birth weight and ADHD symptom severity. These proinflammatory cytokines affect the monoamine system in the brain directly[158,174] and via its effects on the microbiome, creating a mechanistic link between immune function and neurotransmission deficits associated with ADHD. Both child and adult ADHD were associated with the ciliary neurotrophic factor receptor,[173,175] and this provides an important clue in understanding the role of (neuro)inflammation in the development of ADHD, as this factor is important during neurodevelopment by promoting and maintaining hippocampal neurons and modulating serotonergic and cholinergic neurotransmitter systems.[176–179]

CIRCULATING LEVELS OF IMMUNE PARAMETERS RELATE WITH ATTENTION-DEFICIT/ HYPERACTIVITY DISORDER PATHOLOGY

Perinatal stress and early life stress affect infant microbial composition. Effects of stress on gut immune functioning, including intestinal and BBB function, relate to psychiatric disorders such as depression and may similarly contribute to ADHD pathology.[180] Low-grade inflammation and immune activation are known to affect synaptic plasticity and neurogenesis, activating cytokine-producing microglia and affecting neurotransmitter systems. The stress hormone cortisol modulates the ratio of proinflammatory type 1 to antiinflammatory type 2 T-helper cell ratio.[181] Part of cause of ADHD is a deficient HPA functioning (see section on the VN pathway), specifically deficient cortisol response in response to stressors,[182] which may contribute to ADHD symptoms.

Unfortunately, no studies linking specific gut bacterial strains to immune parameters such as the T-helper 1/T-helper 2 (Th1/Th2) balance exist in ADHD. Although, matching inflammatory markers with microbial strains (eg, cytokines) is currently ongoing but complex.[183] Also, in a few studies, the state of the immune function in patients with ADHD is assessed, showing an overall pattern of low-grade inflammation.[178] Some cytokines relate with ADHD pathology. For example, IL-13 and interferon-γ levels were reduced in medicated versus unmedicated patients with ADHD, indicating that pharmacologic treatment intervenes in immune pathology.[184] In unmedicated patients with ADHD, IL-13 levels related with inattention symptoms, IL-16 levels with hyperactivity, and both with errors on a cognitive task measuring motor-coordination and attention.[185] Reaction time variability related with lower TNF-α but higher interferon-γ levels. These task performances reflect behavior seen in patients with ADHD. The relation between inflammatory markers, ADHD symptoms, and cognitive and mental functioning needs to be further tested using large sample sizes, mapping also the interaction between microbial composition and inflammatory markers in this respect.

Are ADHD symptoms observed due to an immune reaction to food? Treatment with elimination diets: clinical observations triggered the idea that adverse behavior as seen in ADHD can (also) be caused by food sensitivity, an immune reaction to food, similar to the allergic reaction seen in atopic diseases.[60] Gut microbes also play a crucial role in food sensitivity through proinflammatory signals that promote T regulatory cells.[186] Exactly which inflammatory signals (triggered by food) that significantly contributes to ADHD pathophysiology remain unclear, as the "typical" immunoglobulin antibody reaction (seen in food allergy) has not been linked to ADHD symptoms.[63] Currently, clinical studies, using oligoantigenic type elimination diets (eg, excluding hyperallergenic foods such as cow's milk and chocolate), show a greater than 40% symptom reduction in a subgroup of affected participants. Smaller effects were observed when eliminating artificial and/or natural salicylates present in, for example, food colorings and preservatives on attention tests and ADHD symptoms.[52,64]

FUTURE DIRECTIONS

ADHD (with its frequent comorbidity with other psychiatric and somatic disorders) places a high burden on patients, their families, and society and cannot be cured. With its persistence into adulthood (in many patients), it is a lifelong condition with high-impact societal consequences (ie, school failure, problems in sustaining personal and work relationships).[187] Clinical management of ADHD requires a significant leap toward understanding disease cause. The discovery of new (putative) microbiome-dependent biological pathways for the onset and persistence of ADHD is one of the objectives here. The identification of novel (microbiome produced) metabolic players will allow the identification of potentially harmful/beneficial compounds involved in (abnormal) neurodevelopment, brain (dys)function, behavioral changes, and the risk of psychiatric disease.

In this review, the authors focus on directional communication, that is, how each individual patient's gut influences the brain, as this promises most insights for establishing biomarkers and novel treatment options. However, for a complete picture of the role of the GBA in causing ADHD, research should also investigate the opposite direction: from the brain to the gut (ie, stress and emotions that influence gut microbiome composition and gastrointestinal function).

Size Does Matter

It is yet to be shown if there is a specific "ADHD microbiome profile," that is, a signature composition of gut microbiota (associated with the disorder) that could be used as a biomarker for ADHD (independently or in interaction with other risk factors such as genetic predisposition).

For all 3 routes described in this review most evidence comes from animal work or small clinical studies. Therefore, more, and larger, clinical studies are needed to establish and confirm their essential role in ADHD pathophysiology. Well-powered studies (eg, following the approaches currently used in Genome Wide Association Studies) should be focused on, first, identifying the bacterial links between the GBA routes (via eg, association studies) and, second, understanding the biological mechanisms of the bacterial taxa involved in each of these pathways in ADHD. Such studies should include detailed (whole genome) sequencing of gut microbiota and information at the (bacterial) metabolic levels combined with behavioral and brain measures (ie, MRI-based).

Everything Is Genetic

It is yet unknown whether or how the hosts' genome modifies microbiome effects. Monozygotic and dizygotic twins have equally similar microbiomes, suggesting the environment may drive familial similarities. However, twins and mother-daughter pairs exhibit more similar microbiome compositions than unrelated individuals, suggesting a genetic influence.[188] Although environmental factors are of importance to ADHD, they have largely been ignored. This may explain some of the inconsistencies in the existing genetic literature. Where gene–environment interactions have been studied, those approaches have not gone beyond candidate-based approaches so far[189] and have not included key factors such as the microbiome, diet, or exercise. A key future step is to use large existing samples to pioneer studies into how the role of gene–environment interaction moderates the links between microbiome and ADHD, taking into account diet and lifestyle.

Gut-Microbiota as Target and Predictor of Treatments

The microbiome is amenable to human intervention (ie, fecal transplant and/or diet), which makes it an attractive candidate for the development of new treatment strategies for psychiatric disorders. Changes in the host's diet and nutrition status can modify its microbial composition and behavior.

It was observed that 3 enterotypes could be associated with different dietary profiles[190,191]: the genus *Prevotella* was found to be adapted to a carbohydrate-dominated metabolism and a vegetarian diet; *Bacteroides*, in turn, was linked to diets that were high in protein and animal-derived products (mostly omnivorous), and microbiota rich in *Firmicutes* (which includes the enterotype Ruminococcus) was strongly associated with a fat-based westernized diet[192] and obesity,[193] even though it seems that species of the same taxonomic group may harbor different metabolic characteristics.[194] Besides the effect of diet, exposure to antibiotics in food or clinical treatments can also have a fast and profound effect in the functioning and composition of the microbiome.

This means that the gut microbiome composition and function could help in (1) enhancing treatment adherence in families reluctant to medicate children and/or in adults unwilling to adhere to treatment and (2) predicting treatment outcomes according to patient subgroups (ie, including specific diets). Depending on the microbiome composition, in combination with the experienced symptoms, behavioral impairments, and perhaps even genetic profile, particular diets can be advised. Such diets target particular nutrient deficiencies that increase neurotransmitter availability or reduce allergic reactions that trigger an immune response that protect against detrimental effects of stress (on microbiome and immune system). Combinations of treatments are also likely to be of effect, such as combining diet with regular physical exercising or behavioral interventions such as mindfulness.[54]

From treatment response it is known that the composition of the human microbiota can change during treatment and also that the microbiota can process medication and thereby affect medication levels and treatment outcome.[195] Gut microbiota can process orally ingested medication before uptake by the gut. This has been demonstrated for several psychotropics, such as the antipsychotic olanzapine,[196,197] commonly prescribed as treatment for schizophrenia, bipolar disorder, and other psychotic disorders. Moreover, recent studies have linked the pharmacokinetics of medication to the gut microbiota.[198–201] If this means that this influence by gut microbiota is a cause for ineffective treatment,[198,202] it could help explain why ADHD medication is not always effective.

SUMMARY

Research on the effects of the gut microbiome, via the GBA in ADHD introduces a novel paradigm and has the potential to set in motion a real conceptual change: neurodevelopmental diseases such as ADHD (and related comorbidities) should no longer be considered brain disorders exclusively, but rather disorders that present as the effect of interactions between the microbiome, host genetics, the gastrointestinal system, and the brain.

REFERENCES

1. Bastiaanssen TFS, Cowan CSM, Claesson MJ, et al. Making sense of… the microbiome in psychiatry. Int J Neuropsychopharmacol 2018. https://doi.org/10.1093/ijnp/pyy067.
2. Vuong HE, Yano JM, Fung TC, et al. The microbiome and host behavior. Annu Rev Neurosci 2017;40:21–49.
3. Cryan JF, Dinan TG. Mind-altering microorganisms: the impact of the gut microbiota on brain and behaviour. Nat Rev Neurosci 2012;13(10):701–12.
4. Gershon MD. Developmental determinants of the independence and complexity of the enteric nervous system. Trends Neurosci 2010;33(10):446–56.

5. Hsiao EY, McBride SW, Hsien S, et al. Microbiota modulate behavioral and physiological abnormalities associated with neurodevelopmental disorders. Cell 2013;155(7):1451–63.
6. Association AP. Diagnostic and statistical manual of mental disorders. 5th edition. Washington, DC: American Psychiatric Association; 2013.
7. Polanczyk G, de Lima MS, Horta BL, et al. The worldwide prevalence of ADHD: a systematic review and metaregression analysis. Am J Psychiatry 2007;164(6): 942–8.
8. Simon V, Czobor P, Balint S, et al. Prevalence and correlates of adult attention-deficit hyperactivity disorder: meta-analysis. Br J Psychiatry 2009;194(3): 204–11.
9. Larsson H, Dilshad R, Lichtenstein P, et al. Developmental trajectories of DSM-IV symptoms of attention-deficit/hyperactivity disorder: genetic effects, family risk and associated psychopathology. J Child Psychol Psychiatry 2011;52(9): 954–63.
10. Willcutt EG. The prevalence of DSM-IV attention-deficit/hyperactivity disorder: a meta-analytic review. Neurotherapeutics 2012;9(3):490–9.
11. Cortese S, Faraone SV, Bernardi S, et al. Gender differences in adult attention-deficit/hyperactivity disorder: results from the National Epidemiologic Survey on Alcohol and Related Conditions (NESARC). J Clin Psychiatry 2016;77(4): e421–8.
12. Quinn PO, Madhoo M. A review of attention-deficit/hyperactivity disorder in women and girls: uncovering this hidden diagnosis. Prim Care Companion CNS Disord 2014;16(3). https://doi.org/10.4088/PCC.13r01596.
13. Chen Q, Hartman CA, Haavik J, et al. Common psychiatric and metabolic comorbidity of adult attention-deficit/hyperactivity disorder: a population-based cross-sectional study. PLoS One 2018;13(9):e0204516.
14. Rommelse NN, Geurts HM, Franke B, et al. A review on cognitive and brain endophenotypes that may be common in autism spectrum disorder and attention-deficit/hyperactivity disorder and facilitate the search for pleiotropic genes. Neurosci Biobehav Rev 2011;35(6):1363–96.
15. Cohen SC, Leckman JF, Bloch MH. Clinical assessment of Tourette syndrome and tic disorders. Neurosci Biobehav Rev 2013;37(6):997–1007.
16. Hart SA, Petrill SA, Willcutt E, et al. Exploring how symptoms of attention-deficit/hyperactivity disorder are related to reading and mathematics performance: general genes, general environments. Psychol Sci 2010;21(11):1708–15.
17. Storebo OJ, Simonsen E. The association between ADHD and antisocial personality disorder (ASPD): a review. J Atten Disord 2016;20(10):815–24.
18. Connor DF, Steeber J, McBurnett K. A review of attention-deficit/hyperactivity disorder complicated by symptoms of oppositional defiant disorder or conduct disorder. J Dev Behav Pediatr 2010;31(5):427–40.
19. van de Glind G, Konstenius M, Koeter MWJ, et al. Variability in the prevalence of adult ADHD in treatment seeking substance use disorder patients: results from an international multi-center study exploring DSM-IV and DSM-5 criteria. Drug Alcohol Depend 2014;134:158–66.
20. Roy A, Oldehinkel AJ, Verhulst FC, et al. Anxiety and disruptive behavior mediate pathways from attention-deficit/hyperactivity disorder to depression. J Clin Psychiatry 2014;75(2):e108–13.
21. Klassen LJ, Katzman MA, Chokka P. Adult ADHD and its comorbidities, with a focus on bipolar disorder. J Affect Disord 2010;124(1–2):1–8.

22. Skirrow C, Asherson P. Emotional lability, comorbidity and impairment in adults with attentiondeficit hyperactivity disorder. J Affect Disord 2013;147(1–3):80–6.

23. Cortese S, Moreira-Maia CR, St Fleur D, et al. Association between ADHD and obesity: a systematic review and meta-analysis. Am J Psychiatry 2016;173(1): 34–43.

24. Hegvik TA, Instanes JT, Haavik J, et al. Associations between attentiondeficit/hyperactivity disorder and autoimmune diseases are modified by sex: a population-based cross-sectional study. Eur Child Adolesc Psychiatry 2018; 27(5):663–75.

25. Faraone SV, Asherson P, Banaschewski T, et al. Attention-deficit/hyperactivity disorder. Nat Rev Dis Primers 2015;1:15020.

26. Faraone SV, Perlis RH, Doyle AE, et al. Molecular genetics of attention-deficit/ hyperactivity disorder. Biol Psychiatry 2005;57(11):1313–23.

27. Faraone SV, Larsson H. Genetics of attention deficit hyperactivity disorder. Mol Psychiatry 2018. https://doi.org/10.1038/s41380-018-0070-0.

28. Franke B, Faraone SV, Asherson P, et al. The genetics of attention deficit/hyperactivity disorder in adults, a review. Mol Psychiatry 2012;17(10):960–87.

29. Gizer IR, Ficks C, Waldman ID. Candidate gene studies of ADHD: a meta-analytic review. Hum Genet 2009;126(1):51–90.

30. Demontis D, Walters RK, Martin J, et al. Discovery of the first genome-wide significant risk loci for attention deficit/hyperactivity disorder. Nat Genet 2018. https://doi.org/10.1038/s41588-018-0269-7.

31. Hoogman M, Bralten J, Hibar DP, et al. Subcortical brain volume differences in participants with attention deficit hyperactivity disorder in children and adults: a cross-sectional mega-analysis. Lancet Psychiatry 2017;4(4):310–9.

32. Cortese S, Kelly C, Chabernaud C, et al. Toward systems neuroscience of ADHD: a meta-analysis of 55 fMRI studies. Am J Psychiatry 2012;169(10): 1038–55.

33. Castellanos FX, Proal E. Large-scale brain systems in ADHD: beyond the prefrontal-striatal model. Trends Cogn Sci 2012;16(1):17–26.

34. Durston S, van Belle J, de Zeeuw P. Differentiating frontostriatal and fronto-cerebellar circuits in attention-deficit/hyperactivity disorder. Biol Psychiatry 2011;69(12):1178–84.

35. Del Campo N, Chamberlain SR, Sahakian BJ, et al. The roles of dopamine and noradrenaline in the pathophysiology and treatment of attention-deficit/hyperactivity disorder. Biol Psychiatry 2011;69(12):e145–57.

36. Hayes DJ, Jupp B, Sawiak SJ, et al. Brain gamma-aminobutyric acid: a neglected role in impulsivity. Eur J Neurosci 2014;39(11):1921–32.

37. Banerjee E, Nandagopal K. Does serotonin deficit mediate susceptibility to ADHD? Neurochem Int 2015;82:52–68.

38. Plichta MM, Scheres A. Ventral-striatal responsiveness during reward anticipation in ADHD and its relation to trait impulsivity in the healthy population: a meta-analytic review of the fMRI literature. Neurosci Biobehav Rev 2014;38: 125–34.

39. Makris N, Biederman J, Monuteaux MC, et al. Towards conceptualizing a neural systemsbased anatomy of attention-deficit/hyperactivity disorder. Dev Neurosci 2009;31(1–2):36–49.

40. Banerjee TD, Middleton F, Faraone SV. Environmental risk factors for attention-deficit hyperactivity disorder. Acta Paediatr 2007;96(9):1269–74.

41. Mill J, Petronis A. Pre- and peri-natal environmental risks for attention-deficit hyperactivity disorder (ADHD): the potential role of epigenetic processes in mediating susceptibility. J Child Psychol Psychiatry 2008;49(10):1020–30.
42. Sciberras E, Mulraney M, Silva D, et al. Prenatal risk factors and the etiology of ADHDReview of existing evidence. Curr Psychiatry Rep 2017;19(1):1.
43. Froehlich TE, Anixt JS, Loe IM, et al. Update on environmental risk factors for attention-deficit/hyperactivity disorder. Curr Psychiatry Rep 2011;13(5):333–44.
44. Kooij JJS, Bijlenga D, Salerno L, et al. Updated European Consensus Statement on diagnosis and treatment of adult ADHD. Eur Psychiatry 2018;56:14–34.
45. Cortese S, Adamo N, Del Giovane C, et al. Comparative efficacy and tolerability of medications for attention-deficit hyperactivity disorder in children, adolescents, and adults: a systematic review and network meta-analysis. Lancet Psychiatry 2018;5(9):727–38.
46. National Institute for Health and Care Excellence. Attention deficit hyperactivity disorder: diagnosis and management. Secondary National Institute for Health and Care Excellence; 2018. Attention deficit hyperactivity disorder: diagnosis and management. Available at: https://www.nice.org.uk/guidance/ng87.
47. Kuczenski R, Segal DS. Effects of methylphenidate on extracellular dopamine, serotonin, and norepinephrine: comparison with amphetamine. J Neurochem 1997;68(5):2032–7.
48. Fredriksen M, Halmoy A, Faraone SV, et al. Long-term efficacy and safety of treatment with stimulants and atomoxetine in adult ADHD: a review of controlled and naturalistic studies. Eur Neuropsychopharmacol 2013;23(6):508–27.
49. Coghill DR, Banaschewski T, Soutullo C, et al. Systematic review of quality of life and functional outcomes in randomized placebo-controlled studies of medications for attentiondeficit/hyperactivity disorder. Eur Child Adolesc Psychiatry 2017;26(11):1283–307.
50. Spencer T, Biederman J, Wilens T, et al. Pharmacotherapy of attention-deficit hyperactivity disorder across the life cycle. J Am Acad Child Adolesc Psychiatry 1996;35(4):409–32.
51. Schwartz S, Correll CU. Efficacy and safety of atomoxetine in children and adolescents with attention-deficit/hyperactivity disorder: results from a comprehensive meta-analysis and metaregression. J Am Acad Child Adolesc Psychiatry 2014;53(2):174–87.
52. Sonuga-Barke EJ, Brandeis D, Cortese S, et al. Nonpharmacological interventions for ADHD: systematic review and meta-analyses of randomized controlled trials of dietary and psychological treatments. Am J Psychiatry 2013;170(3):275–89.
53. De Crescenzo F, Cortese S, Adamo N, et al. Pharmacological and nonpharmacological treatment of adults with ADHD: a meta-review. Evid Based Ment Health 2017;20(1):4–11.
54. Cairncross M, Miller CJ. The effectiveness of mindfulness-based therapies for ADHD: a metaanalytic review. J Atten Disord 2016. https://doi.org/10.1177/1087054715625301.
55. Chandler ML. Psychotherapy for adult attention deficit/hyperactivity disorder: a comparison with cognitive behaviour therapy. J Psychiatr Ment Health Nurs 2013;20(9):814–20.
56. Vidal-Estrada R, Bosch-Munso R, Nogueira-Morais M, et al. Psychological treatment of attention deficit hyperactivity disorder in adults: a systematic review. Actas Esp Psiquiatr 2012;40(3):147–54.

57. Mayer K, Wyckoff SN, Fallgatter AJ, et al. Neurofeedback as a nonpharmaco-logical treatment for adults with attention-deficit/hyperactivity disorder (ADHD): study protocol for a randomized controlled trial. Trials 2015;16:174.

58. Holtmann M, Pniewski B, Wachtlin D, et al. Neurofeedback in children with atten-tiondeficit/hyperactivity disorder (ADHD)–a controlled multicenter study of a non-pharmacological treatment approach. BMC Pediatr 2014;14:202.

59. Chang JP, Su KP, Mondelli V, et al. Omega-3 polyunsaturated fatty acids in youths with attention deficit hyperactivity disorder: a systematic review and meta-analysis of clinical trials and biological studies. Neuropsychopharmacol-ogy 2018;43(3):534–45.

60. Ly V, Bottelier M, Hoekstra PJ, et al. Elimination diets' efficacy and mechanisms in attention deficit hyperactivity disorder and autism spectrum disorder. Eur Child Adolesc Psychiatry 2017;26(9):1067–79.

61. Pelsser LM, Frankena K, Toorman J, et al. Diet and ADHD, reviewing the evi-dence: a systematic review of meta-analyses of double-blind placebo-controlled trials evaluating the efficacy of diet interventions on the behavior of children with ADHD. PLoS One 2017;12(1):e0169277.

62. Dong W, Wang R, Ma LN, et al. Influence of age-related learning and memory capacity of mice: different effects of a high and low caloric diet. Aging Clin Exp Res 2016;28(2):303–11.

63. Pelsser LM, Frankena K, Toorman J, et al. Effects of a restricted elimination diet on the behaviour of children with attention-deficit hyperactivity disorder (INCA study): a randomised controlled trial. Lancet 2011;377(9764):494–503.

64. Nigg JT, Lewis K, Edinger T, et al. Meta-analysis of attention-deficit/hyperactivity disorder or attention-deficit/hyperactivity disorder symptoms, restriction diet, and synthetic food color additives. J Am Acad Child Adolesc Psychiatry 2012;51(1):86–97.e8.

65. Howard AL, Robinson M, Smith GJ, et al. ADHD is associated with a "Western" dietary pattern in adolescents. J Atten Disord 2011;15(5):403–11.

66. Massee LA, Ried K, Pase M, et al. The acute and sub-chronic effects of cocoa flavanols on mood, cognitive and cardiovascular health in young healthy adults: a randomized, controlled trial. Front Pharmacol 2015;6:93.

67. Faraone SV, Antshel KM. Towards an evidence-based taxonomy of nonpharma-cologic treatments for ADHD. Child Adolesc Psychiatr Clin N Am 2014;23(4): 965–72.

68. Singh RK, Chang HW, Yan D, et al. Influence of diet on the gut microbiome and implications for human health. J Transl Med 2017;15(1):73.

69. de Theije CG, Bavelaar BM, Lopes da Silva S, et al. Food allergy and food-based therapies in neurodevelopmental disorders. Pediatr Allergy Immunol 2014;25(3):218–26.

70. Hak E, de Vries TW, Hoekstra PJ, et al. Association of childhood attention-deficit/hyperactivity disorder with atopic diseases and skin infections? A matched case-control study using the General Practice Research Database. Ann Allergy Asthma Immunol 2013;111(2):102–6.e2.

71. Bercik P, Denou E, Collins J, et al. The intestinal microbiota affect central levels of brain-derived neurotropic factor and behavior in mice. Gastroenterology 2011;141(2):599–609, 609.e1-3.

72. Partty A, Kalliomaki M, Wacklin P, et al. A possible link between early probiotic intervention and the risk of neuropsychiatric disorders later in childhood: a ran-domized trial. Pediatr Res 2015;77(6):823–8.

73. Aarts E, Ederveen THA, Naaijen J, et al. Gut microbiome in ADHD and its relation to neural reward anticipation. PLoS One 2017;12(9):e0183509.
74. Bonaz B, Bazin T, Pellissier S. The vagus nerve at the interface of the microbiota-gut-brain axis. Front Neurosci 2018;12:49.
75. Keita AV, Soderholm JD. The intestinal barrier and its regulation by neuroimmune factors. Neurogastroenterol Motil 2010;22(7):718–33.
76. Breit S, Kupferberg A, Rogler G, et al. Vagus nerve as modulator of the brain-gut axis in psychiatric and inflammatory disorders. Front Psychiatry 2018;9:44.
77. Grabauskas G, Owyang C. Plasticity of vagal afferent signaling in the gut. Medicina (Kaunas) 2017;53(2):73–84.
78. Cussotto S, Sandhu KV, Dinan TG, et al. The neuroendocrinology of the microbiota-gut-brain axis: a behavioural perspective. Front Neuroendocrinol 2018;51:80–101.
79. Arneth BM. Gut-brain axis biochemical signalling from the gastrointestinal tract to the central nervous system: gut dysbiosis and altered brain function. Postgrad Med J 2018;94(1114):446–52.
80. Cork SC. The role of the vagus nerve in appetite control: implications for the pathogenesis of obesity. J Neuroendocrinol 2018;30(11):e12643.
81. Agostoni E, Chinnock JE, De Daly MB, et al. Functional and histological studies of the vagus nerve and its branches to the heart, lungs and abdominal viscera in the cat. J Physiol 1957;135(1):182–205.
82. Pimenta FS, Ton AMM, Guerra TO, et al. Unmasking the gut-brain axis: how the microbiota influences brain and behaviour. J Food Microbiology 2018;2(Special issue 1):23–34.
83. Mayer EA. Gut feelings: the emerging biology of gut-brain communication. Nat Rev Neurosci 2011;12(8):453–66.
84. Kaelberer MM, Buchanan KL, Klein ME, et al. A gut-brain neural circuit for nutrient sensory transduction. Science 2018;361(6408). https://doi.org/10.1126/science.aat5236.
85. Han W, Tellez LA, Perkins MH, et al. A neural circuit for gut-induced reward. Cell 2018;175(3):887–8, 665-678.e23.
86. Berthoud HR, Neuhuber WL. Functional and chemical anatomy of the afferent vagal system. Auton Neurosci 2000;85(1–3):1–17.
87. Aston-Jones G, Shipley MT, Chouvet G, et al. Afferent regulation of locus coeruleus neurons: anatomy, physiology and pharmacology. Prog Brain Res 1991;88: 47–75.
88. Van Bockstaele EJ, Peoples J, Telegan P. Efferent projections of the nucleus of the solitary tract to peri-locus coeruleus dendrites in rat brain: evidence for a monosynaptic pathway. J Comp Neurol 1999;412(3):410–28.
89. Krahl SE, Clark KB. Vagus nerve stimulation for epilepsy: a review of central mechanisms. Surg Neurol Int 2012;3(Suppl 4):S255–9.
90. Klarer M, Arnold M, Gunther L, et al. Gut vagal afferents differentially modulate innate anxiety and learned fear. J Neurosci 2014;34(21):7067–76.
91. Nishigaki R, Yokoyama Y, Shimizu Y, et al. Monosodium glutamate ingestion during the development period reduces aggression mediated by the vagus nerve in a rat model of attention deficit-hyperactivity disorder. Brain Res 2018;1690: 40–50.
92. Hida H. The importance of vagus nerve afferent in the formation of emotions in attentiondeficit hyperactivity disorder model rat. Brain Nerve 2016;68(6):633–9 [in Japanese].

93. Bravo JA, Forsythe P, Chew MV, et al. Ingestion of Lactobacillus strain regulates emotional behavior and central GABA receptor expression in a mouse via the vagus nerve. Proc Natl Acad Sci U S A 2011;108(38):16050–5.

94. de Carvalho TD, Wajnsztejn R, de Abreu LC, et al. Analysis of cardiac autonomic modulation of children with attention deficit hyperactivity disorder. Neuropsychiatr Dis Treat 2014;10:613–8.

95. Rash JA, Aguirre-Camacho A. Attention-deficit hyperactivity disorder and cardiac vagal control: a systematic review. Atten Defic Hyperact Disord 2012; 4(4):167–77.

96. Koenig J, Rash JA, Kemp AH, et al. Resting state vagal tone in attention deficit (hyperactivity) disorder: a meta-analysis. World J Biol Psychiatry 2017;18(4): 256–67.

97. Sandgren AM, Brummer RJM. ADHD-originating in the gut? The emergence of a new explanatory model. Med Hypotheses 2018;120:135–45.

98. Sable JJ, Knopf KL, Kyle MR, et al. Attention-deficit hyperactivity disorder reduces automatic attention in young adults. Psychophysiology 2013;50(3): 308–13.

99. Prehn-Kristensen A, Wiesner CD, Baving L. Early gamma-band activity during interference predicts working memory distractibility in ADHD. J Atten Disord 2015;19(11):971–6.

100. Aston-Jones G, Waterhouse B. Locus coeruleus: from global projection system to adaptive regulation of behavior. Brain Res 2016;1645:75–8.

101. Aston-Jones G, Rajkowski J, Cohen J. Role of locus coeruleus in attention and behavioral flexibility. Biol Psychiatry 1999;46(9):1309–20.

102. Clark KB, Smith DC, Hassert DL, et al. Posttraining electrical stimulation of vagal afferents with concomitant vagal efferent inactivation enhances memory storage processes in the rat. Neurobiol Learn Mem 1998;70(3):364–73.

103. Clark KB, Naritoku DK, Smith DC, et al. Enhanced recognition memory following vagus nerve stimulation in human subjects. Nat Neurosci 1999;2(1):94–8.

104. Pena DF, Childs JE, Willett S, et al. Vagus nerve stimulation enhances extinction of conditioned fear and modulates plasticity in the pathway from the ventromedial prefrontal cortex to the amygdala. Front Behav Neurosci 2014;8:327.

105. Suarez AN, Hsu TM, Liu CM, et al. Gut vagal sensory signaling regulates hippocampus function through multi-order pathways. Nat Commun 2018;9(1):2181.

106. Klarer M, Weber-Stadlbauer U, Arnold M, et al. Cognitive effects of subdiaphragmatic vagal deafferentation in rats. Neurobiol Learn Mem 2017;142(Pt B): 190–9.

107. Pliszka SR, McCracken JT, Maas JW. Catecholamines in attention-deficit hyperactivity disorder: current perspectives. J Am Acad Child Adolesc Psychiatry 1996;35(3):264–72.

108. Biederman J, Spencer T. Attention-deficit/hyperactivity disorder (ADHD) as a noradrenergic disorder. Biol Psychiatry 1999;46(9):1234–42.

109. van Kessel SP, Frye AK, El-Gendy AO, et al. Gut bacterial tyrosine decarboxylases restrict the bioavailability of levodopa, the primary treatment in Parkinson's disease. bioRxiv 2018;356246. https://doi.org/10.1101/356246.

110. Clarke G, Stilling RM, Kennedy PJ, et al. Minireview: gut microbiota: the neglected endocrine organ. Mol Endocrinol 2014;28(8):1221–38.

111. Asano Y, Hiramoto T, Nishino R, et al. Critical role of gut microbiota in the production of biologically active, free catecholamines in the gut lumen of mice. Am J Physiol Gastrointest Liver Physiol 2012;303(11):G1288–95.

112. Diaz Heijtz R, Wang S, Anuar F, et al. Normal gut microbiota modulates brain development and behavior. Proc Natl Acad Sci U S A 2011;108(7):3047–52.

113. Wang LJ, Yu YH, Fu ML, et al. Attention deficit-hyperactivity disorder is associated with allergic symptoms and low levels of hemoglobin and serotonin. Sci Rep 2018;8:10229.

114. Hou YW, Xiong P, Gu X, et al. Association of serotonin receptors with attention deficit hyperactivity disorder: a systematic review and meta-analysis. Curr Med Sci 2018;38(3):538–51.

115. Aggarwal S, Mortensen OV. Overview of monoamine transporters. Curr Protoc Pharmacol 2017;79:12, 16 1-12 16 17.

116. Martin CR, Osadchiy V, Kalani A, et al. The brain-gut-microbiome axis. Cell Mol Gastroenterol Hepatol 2018;6(2):133–48.

117. Yano JM, Yu K, Donaldson GP, et al. Indigenous bacteria from the gut microbiota regulate host serotonin biosynthesis. Cell 2015;161(2):264–76.

118. O'Mahony SM, Clarke G, Borre YE, et al. Serotonin, tryptophan metabolism and the brain-gut-microbiome axis. Behav Brain Res 2015;277:32–48.

119. Malinova TS, Dijkstra CD, de Vries HE. Serotonin: a mediator of the gut-brain axis in multiple sclerosis. Mult Scler 2018;24(9):1144–50.

120. de J R De-Paula V, Forlenza AS, Forlenza OV. Relevance of gutmicrobiota in cognition, behaviour and Alzheimer's disease. Pharmacol Res 2018;136:29–34.

121. Kennedy PJ, Cryan JF, Dinan TG, et al. Kynurenine pathway metabolism and the microbiotagut-brain axis. Neuropharmacology 2017;112(Pt B):399–412.

122. Richard DM, Dawes MA, Mathias CW, et al. LTryptophan: basic metabolic functions, behavioral research and therapeutic indications. Int J Tryptophan Res 2009;2:45–60.

123. Clarke G, Grenham S, Scully P, et al. The microbiome-gut-brain axis during early life regulates the hippocampal serotonergic system in a sex-dependent manner. Mol Psychiatry 2013;18(6):666–73.

124. Gao J, Xu K, Liu H, et al. Impact of the gut microbiota on intestinal immunity mediated by tryptophan metabolism. Front Cell Infect Microbiol 2018;8:13.

125. Ghajar A, Aghajan-Nashtaei F, Afarideh M, et al. l-Carnosine as adjunctive therapy in children and adolescents with attention-deficit/hyperactivity disorder: a randomized, double-blind, placebo-controlled clinical trial. J Child Adolesc Psychopharmacol 2018;28(5):331–8.

126. Schur RR, Draisma LW, Wijnen JP, et al. Brain GABA levels across psychiatric disorders: a systematic literature review and meta-analysis of (1) H-MRS studies. Hum Brain Mapp 2016;37(9):3337–52.

127. Satoh H, Suzuki H, Saitow F. Downregulation of dopamine D1-like receptor pathways of GABAergic interneurons in the anterior cingulate cortex of spontaneously hypertensive rats. Neuroscience 2018;394:267–85.

128. Dhakal R, Bajpai VK, Baek KH. Production of gaba (gamma - Aminobutyric acid) by microorganisms: a review. Braz J Microbiol 2012;43(4):1230–41.

129. Sudo N. Microbiome, HPA axis and production of endocrine hormones in the gut. Adv Exp Med Biol 2014;817:177–94.

130. Barrett E, Ross RP, O'Toole PW, et al. gamma-Aminobutyric acid production by culturable bacteria from the human intestine. J Appl Microbiol 2012;113(2):411–7.

131. Feehily C, Karatzas KA. Role of glutamate metabolism in bacterial responses towards acid and other stresses. J Appl Microbiol 2013;114(1):11–24.

132. Janik R, Thomason LAM, Stanisz AM, et al. Magnetic resonance spectroscopy reveals oral Lactobacillus promotion of increases in brain GABA, N-acetyl aspartate and glutamate. Neuroimage 2016;125:988–95.

133. Strandwitz P, Kim KH, Terekhova D, et al. GABA-modulating bacteria of the human gut microbiota. Nat Microbiol 2018. https://doi.org/10.1038/s41564-018-0307-3.

134. Yunes RA, Poluektova EU, Dyachkova MS, et al. GABA production and structure of gadB/gadC genes in Lactobacillus and Bifidobacterium strains from human microbiota. Anaerobe 2016;42:197204.

135. Prehn-Kristensen A, Zimmermann A, Tittmann L, et al. Reduced microbiome alpha diversity in young patients with ADHD. PLoS One 2018;13(7):e0200728.

136. LeBlanc JG, Milani C, de Giori GS, et al. Bacteria as vitamin suppliers to their host: a gut microbiota perspective. Curr Opin Biotechnol 2013;24(2):160–8.

137. Rowland I, Gibson G, Heinken A, et al. Gut microbiota functions: metabolism of nutrients and other food components. Eur J Nutr 2018;57(1):1–24.

138. Ebadi M. Regulation and function of pyridoxal phosphate in CNS. Neurochem Int 1981;3(34):181–205.

139. Dolina S, Margalit D, Malitsky S, et al. Attention-deficit hyperactivity disorder (ADHD) as a pyridoxine-dependent condition: urinary diagnostic biomarkers. Med Hypotheses 2014;82(1):111–6.

140. Landaas ET, Aarsland TI, Ulvik A, et al. Vitamin levels in adults with ADHD. BJPsych Open 2016;2(6):377–84.

141. Aarsland TI, Landaas ET, Hegvik TA, et al. Serum concentrations of kynurenines in adult patients with attention-deficit hyperactivity disorder (ADHD): a case-control study. Behav Brain Funct 2015;11(1):36.

142. Mousain-Bosc M, Roche M, Polge A, et al. Improvement of neurobehavioral disorders in children supplemented with magnesium-vitamin B6. I. Attention deficit hyperactivity disorders. Magnes Res 2006;19(1):46–52.

143. Koh A, De Vadder F, Kovatcheva-Datchary P, et al. From dietary fiber to host physiology: short-chain fatty acids as key bacterial metabolites. Cell 2016;165(6):1332–45.

144. Sherwin E, Rea K, Dinan TG, et al. A gut (microbiome) feeling about the brain. Curr Opin Gastroenterol 2016;32(2):96–102.

145. Sherwin E, Sandhu KV, Dinan TG, et al. May the force be with you: the light and dark sides of the microbiota-gut-brain axis in neuropsychiatry. CNS Drugs 2016;30(11):1019–41.

146. Michel L, Prat A. One more role for the gut: microbiota and blood brain barrier. Ann Transl Med 2016;4(1):15.

147. Kealy J, Greene C, Campbell M. Blood-brain barrier regulation in psychiatric disorders. Neurosci Lett 2018. https://doi.org/10.1016/j.neulet.2018.06.033.

148. Leffa DT, Torres ILS, Rohde LA. A review on the role of inflammation in attention-deficit/hyperactivity disorder. Neuroimmunomodulation 2018;1–6. https://doi.org/10.1159/000489635.

149. Braniste V, Al-Asmakh M, Kowal C, et al. The gut microbiota influences blood-brain barrier permeability in mice. Sci Transl Med 2014;6(263):263ra158.

150. Arentsen T, Qian Y, Gkotzis S, et al. The bacterial peptidoglycan-sensing molecule Pglyrp2 modulates brain development and behavior. Mol Psychiatry 2017;22(2):257–66.

151. Thaiss CA, Zmora N, Levy M, et al. The microbiome and innate immunity. Nature 2016;535(7610):65–74.

152. Macpherson A, Khoo UY, Forgacs I, et al. Mucosal antibodies in inflammatory bowel disease are directed against intestinal bacteria. Gut 1996;38(3):365–75.

153. Christmann BS, Abrahamsson TR, Bernstein CN, et al. Human seroreactivity to gut microbiota antigens. J Allergy Clin Immunol 2015;136(5):1378–86.e1-5.

154. Okun E, Griffioen KJ, Mattson MP. Toll-like receptor signaling in neural plasticity and disease. Trends Neurosci 2011;34(5):269–81.

155. Erny D, Hrabe de Angelis AL, Prinz M. Communicating systems in the body: how microbiota and microglia cooperate. Immunology 2017;150(1):7–15.

156. Bilbo SD, Schwarz JM. The immune system and developmental programming of brain and behavior. Front Neuroendocrinol 2012;33(3):267–86.

157. Kelly JR, Kennedy PJ, Cryan JF, et al. Breaking down the barriers: the gut microbiome, intestinal permeability and stress-related psychiatric disorders. Front Cell Neurosci 2015;9:392.

158. Felger JC, Treadway MT. Inflammation effects on motivation and motor activity: role of dopamine. Neuropsychopharmacology 2017;42(1):216–41.

159. Wang Y, Kasper LH. The role of microbiome in central nervous system disorders. Brain Behav Immun 2014;38:1–12.

160. Moloney RD, Johnson AC, O'Mahony SM, et al. Stress and the microbiota-gut-brain axis in visceral pain: relevance to irritable bowel syndrome. CNS Neurosci Ther 2016;22(2):102–17.

161. Jiang H, Ling Z, Zhang Y, et al. Altered fecal microbiota composition in patients with major depressive disorder. Brain Behav Immun 2015;48:186–94.

162. Evrensel A, Ceylan ME. The gut-brain axis: the missing link in depression. Clin Psychopharmacol Neurosci 2015;13(3):239–44.

163. Miller AH, Raison CL. The role of inflammation in depression: from evolutionary imperative to modern treatment target. Nat Rev Immunol 2016;16(1):22–34.

164. Meltzer A, Van de Water J. The role of the immune system in autism spectrum disorder. Neuropsychopharmacology 2017;42(1):284–98.

165. Miyazaki C, Koyama M, Ota E, et al. Allergic diseases in children with attention deficit hyperactivity disorder: a systematic review and meta-analysis. BMC Psychiatry 2017;17(1):120.

166. Schans JV, Cicek R, de Vries TW, et al. Association of atopic diseases and attentiondeficit/hyperactivity disorder: a systematic review and meta-analyses. Neurosci Biobehav Rev 2017;74(Pt A):139–48.

167. Simpson EL. Comorbidity in atopic dermatitis. Curr Dermatol Rep 2012;1(1):29–38.

168. Strom MA, Silverberg JI. Association between atopic dermatitis and extracutaneous infections in US adults. Br J Dermatol 2017;176(2):495–7.

169. Segman RH, Meltzer A, Gross-Tsur V, et al. Preferential transmission of interleukin-1 receptor antagonist alleles in attention deficit hyperactivity disorder. Mol Psychiatry 2002;7(1):72–4.

170. Drtilkova I, Sery O, Theiner P, et al. Clinical and molecular-genetic markers of ADHD in children. Neuro Endocrinol Lett 2008;29(3):320–7.

171. Lasky-Su J, Neale BM, Franke B, et al. Genome-wide association scan of quantitative traits for attention deficit hyperactivity disorder identifies novel associations and confirms candidate gene associations. Am J Med Genet B Neuropsychiatr Genet 2008;147B(8):1345–54.

172. Lasky-Su J, Anney RJ, Neale BM, et al. Genome-wide association scan of the time to onset of attention deficit hyperactivity disorder. Am J Med Genet B Neuropsychiatr Genet 2008;147B(8):13558.

173. Smith TF, Anastopoulos AD, Garrett ME, et al. Angiogenic, neurotrophic, and inflammatory system SNPs moderate the association between birth weight and ADHD symptom severity. Am J Med Genet B Neuropsychiatr Genet 2014; 165B(8):691–704.
174. Dunn AJ. Effects of cytokines and infections on brain neurochemistry. Clin Neurosci Res 2006;6(1–2):52–68.
175. Ribases M, Hervas A, Ramos-Quiroga JA, et al. Association study of 10 genes encoding neurotrophic factors and their receptors in adult and child attention-deficit/hyperactivity disorder. Biol Psychiatry 2008;63(10):935–45.
176. Ip NY, Yancopoulos GD. Ciliary neurotrophic factor and its receptor complex. Prog Growth Factor Res 1992;4(2):139–55.
177. Peruga I, Hartwig S, Merkler D, et al. Endogenous ciliary neurotrophic factor modulates anxiety and depressive-like behavior. Behav Brain Res 2012; 229(2):325–32.
178. Anand D, Colpo GD, Zeni G, et al. Attention-deficit/hyperactivity disorder and inflammation: what does current knowledge tell us? a systematic review. Front Psychiatry 2017;8:228.
179. Pasquin S, Sharma M, Gauchat JF. Ciliary neurotrophic factor (CNTF): new facets of an old molecule for treating neurodegenerative and metabolic syndrome pathologies. Cytokine Growth Factor Rev 2015;26(5):507–15.
180. Dinan TG, Cryan JF. Microbes, immunity, and behavior: psychoneuroimmunology meets the microbiome. Neuropsychopharmacology 2017;42(1):178–92.
181. Verlaet AA, Noriega DB, Hermans N, et al. Nutrition, immunological mechanisms and dietary immunomodulation in ADHD. Eur Child Adolesc Psychiatry 2014; 23(7):519–29.
182. Raz S, Leykin D. Psychological and cortisol reactivity to experimentally induced stress in adults with ADHD. Psychoneuroendocrinology 2015;60:7–17.
183. Oades RD, Dauvermann MR, Schimmelmann BG, et al. Attention-deficit hyperactivity disorder (ADHD) and glial integrity: S100B, cytokines and kynurenine metabolism-effects of medication. Behav Brain Funct 2010;6:29.
184. Oades RD, Myint AM, Dauvermann MR, et al. Attention-deficit hyperactivity disorder (ADHD) and glial integrity: an exploration of associations of cytokines and kynurenine metabolites with symptoms and attention. Behav Brain Funct 2010; 6:32.
185. Schirmer M, Smeekens SP, Vlamakis H, et al. Linking the human gut microbiome to inflammatory cytokine production capacity. Cell 2016;167(7):1897.
186. Caminero A, Meisel M, Jabri B, et al. Mechanisms by which gut microorganisms influence food sensitivities. Nat Rev Gastroenterol Hepatol 2019;16(1):7–18.
187. Wilens TE, Spencer TJ. Understanding attention-deficit/hyperactivity disorder from childhood to adulthood. Postgrad Med 2010;122(5):97–109.
188. Sandoval-Motta S, Aldana M, Martinez-Romero E, et al. The human microbiome and the missing heritability problem. Front Genet 2017;8:80.
189. Liang S, Wu X, Jin F. Gut-brain psychology: rethinking psychology from the microbiota-gutbrain axis. Front Integr Neurosci 2018;12:33.
190. Losasso C, Eckert EM, Mastrorilli E, et al. Assessing the influence of vegan, vegetarian and omnivore oriented westernized dietary styles on human gut microbiota: a cross sectional study. Front Microbiol 2018;9:317.
191. Wu GD, Compher C, Chen EZ, et al. Comparative metabolomics in vegans and omnivores reveal constraints on diet-dependent gut microbiota metabolite production. Gut 2016;65(1):63–72.

192. De Filippo C, Cavalieri D, Di Paola M, et al. Impact of diet in shaping gut micro-biota revealed by a comparative study in children from Europe and rural Africa. Proc Natl Acad Sci U S A 2010;107(33):14691–6.
193. Ley RE, Turnbaugh PJ, Klein S, et al. Microbial ecology: human gut microbes associated with obesity. Nature 2006;444(7122):1022–3.
194. De Filippis F, Pellegrini N, Vannini L, et al. High-level adherence to a Mediterra-nean diet beneficially impacts the gut microbiota and associated metabolome. Gut 2016;65(11):1812–21.
195. Bisanz JE, Spanogiannopoulos P, Pieper LM, et al. How to determine the role of the microbiome in drug disposition. Drug Metab Dispos 2018;46(11):1588–95.
196. Morgan AP, Crowley JJ, Nonneman RJ, et al. The antipsychotic olanzapine inter-acts with the gut microbiome to cause weight gain in mouse. PLoS One 2014; 9(12):e115225.
197. Davey KJ, Cotter PD, O'Sullivan O, et al. Antipsychotics and the gut micro-biome: olanzapineinduced metabolic dysfunction is attenuated by antibiotic administration in the rat. Transl Psychiatry 2013;3:e309.
198. Choi MS, Yu JS, Yoo HH, et al. The role of gut microbiota in the pharmacoki-netics of antihypertensive drugs. Pharmacol Res 2018;130:164–71.
199. Wilson ID, Nicholson JK. Gut microbiome interactions with drug metabolism, ef-ficacy, and toxicity. Transl Res 2017;179:204–22.
200. Kim JK, Choi MS, Jeong JJ, et al. Effect of probiotics on pharmacokinetics of orally administered acetaminophen in mice. Drug Metab Dispos 2018;46(2): 122–30.
201. Yoo DH, Kim IS, Van Le TK, et al. Gut microbiota-mediated drug interactions be-tween lovastatin and antibiotics. Drug Metab Dispos 2014;42(9):1508–13.
202. Li H, Jia W. Cometabolism of microbes and host: implications for drug meta-bolism and druginduced toxicity. Clin Pharmacol Ther 2013;94(5):574–81.

Improving Mental Health for the Mother-Infant Dyad by Nutrition and the Maternal Gut Microbiome

Beatriz Peñalver Bernabé, PhD[a,b],
Lisa Tussing-Humphreys, PhD, MS, RD[b], Hannah S. Rackers, MPH[c],
Lauren Welke, MS[d], Alina Mantha, RD[e], Mary C. Kimmel, MD[c,*]

KEYWORDS

- Nutrition • Gut microbiome • Pregnancy • Postpartum • Depression • Anxiety
- Stress

KEY POINTS

- Several studies linked nutritional composition and perinatal depression.
- The gut microbiome is a mediator between nutrient intake and the brain through the brain-gut axis.
- Dietary patterns, macronutrients, and micronutrients can alter and be altered by gut microbes and are associated with differences in microbial composition.
- Perinatal mood and anxiety disorders (PMAD) in relation to nutrition is better understood when the microbiome is included.
- Gut microbial composition holds promise to direct dietary interventions for PMAD.

INTRODUCTION

Many interventions are aimed at supporting mental health and nutrition during the perinatal period (pregnancy and up to 1 year after childbirth) to improve maternal and child health outcomes. Perinatal mood and anxiety disorders (PMAD) are common, with an

Disclosure Statement: Dr M.C. Kimmel has received support from Sage Therapeutics to speak about perinatal depression. The rest of the authors have nothing to disclose.
[a] Department of Surgery, Microbiome Center, University of Chicago, 5841 S. Maryland Street, Chicago, IL 60637, USA; [b] Division of Academic Internal Medicine, Department of Medicine, Institute for Health Research and Policy Cancer Center, University of Illinois at Chicago, 1747 W. Roosevelt Road, Chicago, IL 60608, USA; [c] Department of Psychiatry, UNC School of Medicine Campus Box 7160, Chapel Hill, NC 27599-7160, USA; [d] Department of Kinesiology and Nutrition, University of Illinois at Chicago, 1919 W. Taylor Street, Chicago, IL 60612, USA; [e] Department of Maternal and Child Health, UNC Gillings School of Global Public Health, 401 Rosenau Hall, CB #7445, Chapel Hill, NC 27599-7445, USA
* Corresponding author.
E-mail address: mary_kimmel@med.unc.edu

Gastroenterol Clin N Am 48 (2019) 433–445
https://doi.org/10.1016/j.gtc.2019.04.007
0889-8553/19/© 2019 Elsevier Inc. All rights reserved.

estimated prevalence of 10% to 20% for severe depression[1] and up to 39% for anxiety disorders, including generalized anxiety, obsessions and compulsions, and exacerbated or new-onset posttraumatic stress.[2] The microbiota (a community of bacteria, viruses, fungi, and protists) that reside in our gut may be a key factor in the relationship between diet and mental health during pregnancy that operates through the gut-brain axis.[3] The gut-brain axis entails complex nonlinear bidirectional interactions between the gut microbiome and the neurologic, endocrine, and immune systems. Nutritional interventions hold potential to prevent and treat PMAD through the regulation of the maternal gut microbiome.

Dietary requirements evolve during the perinatal period to adequately support development of the placenta and fetus while maintaining maternal health through pregnancy and post-delivery.[4] Although malnutrition has been associated with negative effects on maternal mental health and child cognitive development and for the child's development of neuropsychiatric diseases,[5] overnutrition and maternal obesity are also associated with negative outcomes.[6] Maternal mental health is also a factor underlying nutritional status in pregnancy. Anhedonia may decrease motivation to prepare balanced meals, or anxiety and stress might alter appetite or shift intake to nutrient-poor high saturated fat and high sugar diets.[7] The relationship between PMAD and nutrition is difficult to study due to both being multifactorial.[8] The gut microbiome may mediate host-environment interactions that relate diet and PMAD. The gut microbiota interfaces with the host immune system and is involved in the production and metabolism of nutrients physiologically relevant to mental health, such as vitamins, tryptophan, and short chain fatty acids (SCFAs).[9,10] Precision nutrition allows for consideration of these factors and complex interactions resulting from the perinatal period's unique nutritional and physiologic, endocrine, immune, and host microbiome changes.[11] In this review, we examine dynamic perinatal nutritional needs, associations with PMAD, and mediating effects of the gut microbiota. We discuss examples of micronutrients, macronutrients, and dietary patterns and their implications for PMAD, and we review precision nutrition, the utility of prebiotics and probiotics, and future directions for research and treatment for PMAD.

MICRONUTRIENTS
Iron

Iron provides an example of the complexity of tailoring recommendations in the perinatal period. In the second and third trimesters, maternal dietary iron requirements double to support growth of the placenta and fetus, expansion of maternal red blood cells, and increased placental iron transfer for fetal storage.[12] Yet, maternal iron deficiency (ID) remains a public health problem in the United States, with 30% of pregnant women experiencing ID in the third trimester.[13] Iron is a cofactor in the synthesis of tyrosine, a precursor to the dopamine and norepinephrine, and tryptophan.[14] Dysregulation of these neurotransmitters has been implicated in the development of depression, suggesting a role for iron in maintaining mood.[15] A meta-analysis of nonpregnant adults found an inverse relationship between dietary iron intake and depression,[16] and observational studies have found maternal ID and iron deficiency anemia (IDA) were associated with perinatal depression.[17,18]

Germ-free rats have been shown to have reduced capacity to absorb, store, and mobilize iron compared with conventional rats.[19] Research suggests that ID, IDA, and luminal iron excess may affect gut microbiota and their metabolic activity. In an animal model, ID was associated with lower microbial diversity and decreased SCFA production that was partially restored with iron supplementation.[20] While in a human trial, iron supplementation had no effect on the abundance of bacterial groups or bacterial metabolic activity (ie, SCFA production).[21] SCFAs are products from the fermentation of nondigestible carbohydrates that are associated with reduced inflammation and improved general mood. In another human study, the effects of iron supplementation on the microbiota were dependent on the host gut inflammatory status at baseline.[22] In children with ID and underlying gut inflammation, iron supplementation was associated with a relative increase in Enterobacteriaceae and decrease in the genus Lactobacilli that was accompanied by increased gut inflammation. Together these studies suggest that the microbial metabolic milieu associated with an excess or dearth of iron could lead to several physiologic alterations (eg, gut barrier dysfunction, immune activation, and hypothalamic-pituitary-adrenal [HPA] axis dysfunction) that affect mood. Despite known dynamic changes of pregnancy that impact iron levels, no studies have examined microbiome-mediated effects of ID or luminal iron excess on mental health in pregnancy or postpartum.

Vitamin D

During pregnancy, vitamin D is required for bone mineralization, maintaining balance of calcium and phosphorus, immune function, managing oxidative stress, placental development, and glucose management.[23] Vitamin D deficiency has been implicated in perinatal depression. In a systematic review, most studies showed an association between circulating vitamin D levels and depression during pregnancy and postpartum.[24] One randomized controlled trial of pregnant women found that a dose of 2000 IU of vitamin D3 reduce depressive symptoms as determined by the Edinburgh Perinatal Depression Scale at the end of pregnancy and through 8 weeks postpartum.[25]

The maternal microbiota may again be an important factor linking vitamin D to PMAD. A systematic review from animal and human studies during pregnancy identify that lower levels of dietary vitamin D and/or lower measured circulating vitamin D was associated with alterations in specific taxa,[26] but results were not reproducible between studies. A study of more than 900 infants showed that Bifidobacterium species were less abundant in vitamin D–deficient infants.[27] In the general population, the genus Bifidobacterium is inversely correlated with depressive symptoms,[28] and Bifidobacterium strains have been shown to reduce depressive symptoms in humans.[29] Adequate vitamin D levels may promote the growth and maintenance of anti-inflammatory bacteria, for example, Bifidobacterium,[30] whereas low levels may promote proinflammatory bacteria as evidenced by findings of increased circulating lipopolysaccharide (LPS), a proinflammatory bacterial byproduct, when vitamin D levels are low.[31] These associations among vitamin D levels, PMAD, and microbial composition suggest proinflammatory microbiota as a mechanism.

Folic Acid

Folic acid can prevent fetal neural tube defects and is required for the metabolism and synthesis of neurotransmitters and for healthy central nervous system (CNS) function.[32] Low folic acid intake is associated with increased levels of blood homocysteine whose concentrations are linked to mental health disorders, including depression.[33] Importantly, women who exhibit a mutation in the enzyme that transforms folic acid into its active form, L-methyl folate, have an increased risk of depression postpartum.[34] Although one observational study reported lower plasma folate levels in pregnant women with depression, no association was observed with postpartum depression.[35]

Commensal strains of Lactobacillus and Bifidobacterium synthesize vitamins, including folic acid, that can be absorbed and used by the host.[36] A reduction in the abundance of these bacteria could have an effect on host folate availability that negatively impacts oxidative stress, inflammation, and ultimately, mental health. Supplementation with a probiotic that contained *Bifidobacterium, Lactobacillus,* and *Streptococcus* species increased circulating levels of folic acid and vitamin B12, and decreased homocysteine levels in a clinical trial.[37] Animal studies have also shown a modest effect of folic acid supplementation on the composition, structure, and transcriptional profile of microbiome.[38] More studies are needed to understand the role of the microbiome in folic acid synthesis and its effects on host physical and mental health status, particularly during the perinatal period when folic acid needs are high,[39] the composition of the microbiota naturally shifts,[40] and there is an inherent increase in oxidative stress.[41]

MACRONUTRIENTS
Digestible and Nondigestible Carbohydrates

To support the rapid growth and glucose needs of the developing fetus, the recommended daily allowance for carbohydrate in pregnancy increases from 130 (nonpregnant) to 175 g/d and 25 to 28 g/d of dietary fiber.[42] Most reproductive-age women in the United States meet or exceed the general carbohydrate recommendation; although despite the multiple benefits of fiber during pregnancy,[43] mean fiber intake remains far below recommendations at 15 g/d.[44] Results are inconsistent regarding an association between dietary fiber and mood. One study of fiber intake from vegetables and fruits showed a negative association with depressive symptoms.[45] Conversely, in a population-based study of more than 10,000 adults, Seo and Je[46] observed no differences in mean fiber intake in men and women with and without depression. Discrepancies may be associated with the differing dietary trends or with methods used to assess depressive symptoms and diet.

Individual microbiome composition and structure may impact dietary intake and depressive symptoms. Some of the commensal microorganisms that reside in our gut (eg, *Akkermansia muciniphila, Ruminococcus obeum, Faecalibacterium prausnitzii*) can degrade fiber into SCFA, such as acetic, propionic and butyric acid.[47] SCFAs can have local and systemic effects through direct consumption by the host cells or by binding host cellular receptors.[48] Binding of SCFAs to their specific receptors can also reduce chronic inflammation,[49] which is a common hallmark of general and perinatal depression. Several reports suggest that butyrate might have antidepressantlike characteristics.[50] However, blood concentrations of SCFAs were not found to be different in patients with depression versus controls who consumed similar amounts of dietary fiber.[51] Animal models have shown that administration of SCFAs during pregnancy, and continued for pups after birth, led to alterations in the pups' intestinal microbiome while decreasing virus-induced inflammation.[52] This indicates that SCFA intake and production levels during pregnancy may impact the immune system of the offspring as well.

Fat

Dietary fat intake recommendations remain at 20% to 35% of total calories during the perinatal period.[42] Dietary fat is needed to support the growing fetus[53] and to promote optimal macronutrient content of breast milk during lactation.[54]

Saturated fatty acids

Despite their importance, diets high in saturated fatty acids (SFAs) can induce hyperinsulinemia, systemic inflammation, HPA-axis dysfunction, and depressionlike symptoms in animal models.[55] In humans, there is evidence that higher intake of SFAs is associated with HPA-axis disturbances linked to depression.[56] The negative effect of SFAs on mental health may be mediated by the microbiome. In preclinical and clinical studies, diets high in SFAs increased the relative abundance of gram-negative bacteria,[57] including the sulfur-reducing bacterium *Bilophila wadsworthia*, which are associated with increased inflammation, epithelial permeability,[58] and systemic endotoxemia. *B wadsworthia* metabolizes taurine-conjugated bile acids to hydrogen sulfide that can activate proinflammatory pathways.[59] In a mouse model, SFA diet increased LPS translocation more than unsaturated fatty acid diet, induced metabolic endotoxemia, and caused a shift in microbial composition (including decreased *A muciniphila*).[60] *A muciniphila* has been associated with decreased inflammation[61] and decreased anxiety and depressionlike behavior in mice.[62] In animals, *Akkermansia* has been shown to increase during pregnancy and is influenced by maternal dietary fat intake before and during pregnancy.[63] The effect of pregnancy and dietary fat on *Akkermansia* in humans and the relationship to maternal mental health remains unknown.

n-3 polyunsaturated fatty acids

The n-3 polyunsaturated fatty acids (n-3 PUFAs) are essential fatty acids that can be obtained only from the diet, specifically marine-sourced foods, fortified dairy products, canola oil, walnuts, and flaxseed.[64] Essential fatty acids are especially abundant in neuronal membranes, which play an important role in neuronal signal transmission, receptor function, and neurotransmitter uptake.[64] Docosahexaenoic acid (DHA) is the most abundant n-3 PUFA in the brain and is integral to membrane fluidity and serotonin sensitivity.[65] The n-3 PUFAs may also play an important role in controlling brain inflammation,[66] but most studies testing the effect of n-3 PUFA supplementation on PMAD have not provided strong evidence.[67] In a systematic review, Trujillo and colleagues[68] found no effect of circulating n-3 fatty acids on perinatal depression and conflicting results for the association of circulating DHA and fatty acid ratios (n-6 to n-3 ratio) with antenatal depression. Existing evidence is limited in that most studies tested isolated fatty acid supplements rather than the impact of increased consumption of n-3 PUFA-containing foods, which may be more bioavailable.

Supplementation with n-3 PUFAs has been associated with altered microbiota, with increases of some species of Lachnospiraceae and Bacteroidetes in conjunction with a decrease in *Faecalibacterium*.[69] As with SFAs, the relationship among PUFAs, perinatal depression, and maternal microbiome needs to be established.

Protein

Protein needs increase in pregnancy from 0.8 g/kg per day to 1.1 g/kg per day[42] to support fetal growth, including enzyme and collagen production and protein accretion in maternal tissues, including the placenta.[70] Most pregnant women in high-income countries meet or exceed protein needs,[70] but certain groups of women should be monitored for adequate intake, including those who are vegetarian and vegan. The CNS requires several amino acids from protein foods to function optimally,[71] for example, amino acids tryptophan, tyrosine, histidine, and arginine, which are essential for neurotransmitter production.[72]

Tryptophan

Some foods, such as walnuts, have been shown to beneficially influence gut microbial tryptophan pathways that lead to the production of serotonin.[73] Several studies have shown that tryptophan depletion has an effect on mood likely through production of the neurotransmitter, serotonin.[74] In the general population, circulating tryptophan levels are lower in people with depression than nondepressed.[75] In pregnancy, the concentration of tryptophan decreases as the pregnancy progresses, and the depletion is more pronounced in the third trimester.[76] During pregnancy and postpartum, tryptophan levels may also be associated with mood disorders.

Some commensal bacteria, such as *Bacteroides fragilis,* can consume tryptophan as an energy source, thus reducing the available tryptophan in the gut milieu that could be converted into serotonin.[77] Large ratios of kynurenine to tryptophan are associated with perinatal depression and are responsible for a reduced serotonin concentration in the gut. Kynurenine is one of the initial byproducts of the tryptophan metabolism, whose production reduces the rates of the production of serotonin. Supplementation with the probiotic *Lactobacillus johnsonii* in an animal model resulted in lower circulating kynurenine and increases in serotonin levels, indicating a shifting tryptophan metabolism from the kynurenine pathway to serotonin metabolism.[78] Moreover, transplantation from microbiota of depressed patients into healthy rats led to dysregulation of tryptophan metabolism.[51]

DIETARY PATTERNS

Although individual micronutrients and macronutrients can be associated with perinatal depression and the gut microbiome, the interactions between these factors may impact PMAD, as well as warranting investigation of dietary patterns. Several studies have examined associations between dietary patterns and perinatal mood. Consuming an unhealthy diet (ie, refined grains, sweets, energy drinks, fast foods), compared with a healthy diet (ie, fruits, vegetables, fish, whole grains), associated with increased depressive symptoms at 32 gestational weeks.[79] Diets rich in fish, vegetables, plant-based proteins, and nutrients have been associated with decreased risk of antenatal depressive symptoms compared with diets of processed foods and foods high in sodium, saturated fat, trans-fat, and added sugar. Diet quality and inflammation potential have been associated with increased perinatal depressive symptoms[80,81]; however, these relationships may reflect that those who are depressed simply tend to choose less healthy foods. Observational[82,83] and interventional[84,85] studies have demonstrated that adherence to a Mediterranean diet, rich in whole fruits, vegetables, whole grains, fiber, olive oil, and low in red meat, dairy, and processed foods, was associated with decreased depression and depressive symptoms in nonpregnant adults. However, no studies have examined the association of a Mediterranean diet with PMAD or tested the effect of dietary interventions on the prevention and treatment of PMAD.

Dietary patterns show differential effects on the microbiome. Increasing evidence shows the effects of a Western diet and Mediterranean diet on CNS function and mood may be mediated through the microbiome.[86] Consumption of Western-style high-fat diet is associated with decreased gut microbial diversity,[87,88] decreased relative abundance of *Bifidobacteria* and SCFA-producing bacteria like the genus *Roseburia,*[89,90] and increased *Alistipes,* which has been shown to be enriched in the guts of persons with major depressive disorder.[91] Furthermore, consumption of a Western diet is associated with increased levels in the circulating LPS.[92] Transplantation of high-fat diet donor microbiota decreased microbial diversity and gut barrier function in recipient animals; increased circulating endotoxin, immune activation, and systemic and neuro-inflammation; and increased anxietylike behavior, demonstrating microbiome-mediated effects of diet on neuro-psychiatric function in an animal model.[87] In human studies, consuming a Mediterranean diet was associated with increased relative abundance of SCFA-producing bacteria including the genus *Roseburia* and species *F prausnitzii,*[93] increased circulating and stool SCFAs,[88] and decreased systemic inflammation and oxidative stress.[94] These findings suggest that manipulation of the microbiome with diet could affect mental health and PMAD.

PRECISION NUTRITION TO PREVENT AND TREAT PERINATAL MOOD DISORDERS

Despite the importance of timely and effective treatments for PMAD, many women will not be identified and only 3% to 5% of women achieve remission, which highlights the need for new avenues of identification and treatment.[95] This review has identified that certain nutrients and dietary patterns are associated with mood in pregnancy and that the effects of maternal nutrient availability and nutritional status on PMAD may be mediated through the gut microbiome. The gut microbiota is dynamic in the perinatal period[96] an effect that is likely related to individual endocrine, neurologic, and immune changes that accompany pregnancy. Thus, individual fluctuations may shift nutrient bioavailability and the production of diet-derived microbial metabolites that are relevant to PMAD.

Microbial structure and function may serve as biomarkers of risk for PMAD as well as inform dietary recommendations to ensure optimal maternal and fetal health requiring a precision nutrition approach rather than universal recommendations. Zeevi and colleagues[97] recently demonstrated clinical implementation of precision nutrition. Researchers used patient biological information (eg, genetics, epigenetics, transcript and protein levels, and microbial transcript abundance) and clinical metadata to construct an algorithm that was able to predict the most adequate personalized diet for controlling glycemic index.[97] Although the current cost of generating such an extensive phenotype (eg, genome, epigenome, microbiome) may not be clinically feasible, computational approaches, such as machine-learning methods, could be used to integrate numerous factors to predict the risk of PMAD and positively impact mental health outcomes for mother and child.

Prebiotic and probiotic supplementation to treat mood disorders in pregnancy is an active area of research. Animal studies have indicated that prebiotics such as fructo-oligosaccharide and xylo-oligosaccharide decreased anxietylike behavior.[3] Additional research has shown that probiotics may decrease anxiety and depressive symptoms. Administration of *Lactobacillus rhamnosus* HN001 during pregnancy decreased depressive symptoms in a randomized, double-blind, placebo-controlled trial.[98] Probiotic supplements likely need to be tailored to individual characteristics to ensure efficacy and microbial establishment. More research is required to ascertain suitable prebiotics and/or probiotic strains and the appropriate dosing for preventing and treating disease.

The antimicrobial effect of antidepressants is another important consideration when investigating treatments for PMAD involving the gut microbiota.[99] Recently, Karine de Sousa and colleagues[100] demonstrated in vitro that fluoxetine, a selective serotonin reuptake inhibitor, could reduce the abundance of resistant inflammatory strains of *Escherichia coli*, *Staphylococcus aureus*, and *Pseudomonas aeruginosa*. Furthermore, metabolism of antidepressants by the microbiota may impact the efficacy and dose, which is particularly relevant as physiologic changes of pregnancy alter drug metabolism and require dose adjustments.

To conclude, the perinatal period is accompanied by dynamic shifts in the gut microbiome, immune and endocrine systems, and maternal nutritional requirements that interface to effect maternal mental health and child neurodevelopment. This review has identified research that provides examples of how micronutrient, macronutrient, and dietary patterns are impacted by the gut microbial community. Future research should strive to use systems biology approaches to integrate host and microbial characteristics to assess risk for PMAD and to develop nutritional plans to promote mental health for mother and the developing child.

REFERENCES

1. Gavin NI, Gaynes BN, Lohr KN, et al. Perinatal depression: a systematic review of prevalence and incidence. Obstet Gynecol 2005;106(5, Part 1):1071–83.
2. Meltzer-Brody S, Howard LM, Bergink V, et al. Postpartum psychiatric disorders. Nat Rev Dis Primer 2018;4:18022.
3. Rackers HS, Thomas S, Williamson K, et al. Emerging literature in the microbiota-brain axis and perinatal mood and anxiety disorders. Psychoneuroendocrinology 2018;95:86–96.
4. Butte NF, King JC. Energy requirements during pregnancy and lactation. Public Health Nutr 2005;8(7a). https://doi.org/10.1079/PHN2005793.
5. Lindsay KL, Buss C, Wadhwa PD, et al. The interplay between nutrition and stress in pregnancy: implications for fetal programming of brain development. Biol Psychiatry 2018. https://doi.org/10.1016/j.biopsych.2018.06.021.
6. Edlow AG. Maternal obesity and neurodevelopmental and psychiatric disorders in offspring. Prenat Diagn 2017;37(1):95–110.
7. Hurley KM, Caulfield LE, Sacco LM, et al. Psychosocial influences in dietary patterns during pregnancy. J Am Diet Assoc 2005;105(6):963–6.
8. Ferguson LR, De Caterina R, Görman U, et al. Guide and position of the international society of nutrigenetics/nutrigenomics on personalised nutrition: part 1 - fields of precision nutrition. J Nutr Nutr 2016;9(1):12–27.
9. Dinan TG, Cryan JF. Microbes, immunity, and behavior: psychoneuroimmunology meets the microbiome. Neuropsychopharmacology 2017;42(1):178–92.
10. Holzer P, Farzi A. Neuropeptides and the microbiota-gut-brain axis. In: Lyte M, Cryan JF, editors. Microbial endocrinology: the microbiota-gut-brain axis in health and disease, vol. 817. New York: Springer New York; 2014. p. 195–219.
11. Ghaemi MS, DiGiulio DB, Contrepois K, et al. Multiomics modeling of the immunome, transcriptome, microbiome, proteome and metabolome adaptations during human pregnancy. Bioinformatics 2018. https://doi.org/10.1093/bioinformatics/bty537.
12. Kominiarek MA, Rajan P. Nutrition recommendations in pregnancy and lactation. Med Clin North Am 2016;100(6):1199–215.
13. Mei Z, Cogswell ME, Looker AC, et al. Assessment of iron status in US pregnant women from the National Health and Nutrition Examination Survey (NHANES), 1999–2006. Am J Clin Nutr 2011;93(6):1312–20.
14. Beard JL. Iron biology in immune function, muscle metabolism and neuronal functioning. J Nutr 2001;131(2):568S–80S.
15. Richardson A, Heath A-L, Haszard J, et al. Higher body iron is associated with greater depression symptoms among young adult men but not women: observational data from the daily life study. Nutrients 2015;7(8):6055–72.
16. Li Z, Li B, Song X, et al. Dietary zinc and iron intake and risk of depression: a meta-analysis. Psychiatry Res 2017;251:41–7.
17. Dama M, Van Lieshout RJ, Mattina G, et al. Iron deficiency and risk of maternal depression in pregnancy: an observational study. J Obstet Gynaecol Can 2018; 40(6):698–703.
18. Wassef A, Nguyen QD, St-André M. Anaemia and depletion of iron stores as risk factors for postpartum depression: a literature review. J Psychosom Obstet Gynecol 2018;1–10. https://doi.org/10.1080/0167482X.2018.1427725.

19. Reddy BS. Studies on the mechanism of calcium and magnesium absorption in germfree rats. Arch Biochem Biophys 1972;149(1):15–21.
20. Dostal A, Chassard C, Hilty FM, et al. Iron depletion and repletion with ferrous sulfate or electrolytic iron modifies the composition and metabolic activity of the gut microbiota in rats. J Nutr 2012;142(2):271–7.
21. Dostal A, Lacroix C, Pham VT, et al. Iron supplementation promotes gut microbiota metabolic activity but not colitis markers in human gut microbiota-associated rats. Br J Nutr 2014;111(12):2135–45.
22. Zimmermann MB, Harrington M, Villalpando S, et al. Nonheme-iron absorption in first-degree relatives is highly correlated: a stable-isotope study in mother-child pairs. Am J Clin Nutr 2010;91(3):802–7.
23. Wei SQ. Vitamin D and pregnancy outcomes. Curr Opin Obstet Gynecol 2014; 26(6):438–47.
24. Aghajafari F, Letourneau N, Mahinpey N, et al. Vitamin D deficiency and antenatal and postpartum depression: a systematic review. Nutrients 2018; 10(4):478.
25. Vaziri F, Nasiri S, Tavana Z, et al. A randomized controlled trial of vitamin D supplementation on perinatal depression: in Iranian pregnant mothers. BMC Pregnancy Childbirth 2016;16(1):239.
26. Waterhouse M, Hope B, Krause L, et al. Vitamin D and the gut microbiome: a systematic review of in vivo studies. Eur J Nutr 2018. https://doi.org/10.1007/s00394-018-1842-7.
27. Talsness CE, Penders J, Jansen EHJM, et al. Influence of vitamin D on key bacterial taxa in infant microbiota in the KOALA Birth Cohort Study. In: Taneja V, editor. PLoS One 2017;12(11):e0188011.
28. Aizawa E, Tsuji H, Asahara T, et al. Possible association of *Bifidobacterium* and *Lactobacillus* in the gut microbiota of patients with major depressive disorder. J Affect Disord 2016;202:254–7.
29. Pinto-Sanchez MI, Hall GB, Ghajar K, et al. Probiotic *Bifidobacterium longum* NCC3001 reduces depression scores and alters brain activity: a pilot study in patients with irritable bowel syndrome. Gastroenterology 2017;153(2): 448–59.e8.
30. Khokhlova EV, Smeianov VV, Efimov BA, et al. Anti-inflammatory properties of intestinal Bifidobacterium strains isolated from healthy infants. Microbiol Immunol 2012;56(1):27–39.
31. Villa CR, Taibi A, Chen J, et al. Colonic *Bacteroides* are positively associated with trabecular bone structure and programmed by maternal vitamin D in male but not female offspring in an obesogenic environment. Int J Obes 2018;42(4):696–703.
32. Bottiglieri T. Folate, vitamin B12, and neuropsychiatric disorders. Nutr Rev 1996; 54(12):382–90.
33. Bjelland I, Tell GS, Vollset SE, et al. Folate, vitamin B12, homocysteine, and the MTHFR 677C→T polymorphism in anxiety and depression: the Hordaland Homocysteine Study. Arch Gen Psychiatry 2003;60(6):618.
34. Lewis SJ, Araya R, Leary S, et al. Folic acid supplementation during pregnancy may protect against depression 21 months after pregnancy, an effect modified by MTHFR C677T genotype. Eur J Clin Nutr 2012;66(1):97–103.
35. Chong MFF, Wong JXY, Colega M, et al. Relationships of maternal folate and vitamin B12 status during pregnancy with perinatal depression: The GUSTO study. J Psychiatr Res 2014;55:110–6.

36. Rossi M, Amaretti A, Raimondi S. Folate production by probiotic bacteria. Nutrients 2011;3(1):118–34.

37. Valentini L, Pinto A, Bourdel-Marchasson I, et al. Impact of personalized diet and probiotic supplementation on inflammation, nutritional parameters and intestinal microbiota - The "RISTOMED project": randomized controlled trial in healthy older people. Clin Nutr Edinb Scotl 2015;34(4):593–602.

38. Hibberd MC, Wu M, Rodionov DA, et al. The effects of micronutrient deficiencies on bacterial species from the human gut microbiota. Sci Transl Med 2017; 9(390):eaal4069.

39. Greenberg JA, Bell SJ, Guan Y, et al. Folic acid supplementation and pregnancy: more than just neural tube defect prevention. Rev Obstet Gynecol 2011;4(2):52–9.

40. Koren O, Goodrich JK, Cullender TC, et al. Host remodeling of the gut microbiome and metabolic changes during pregnancy. Cell 2012;150(3):470–80.

41. Toescu V, Nuttall SL, Martin U, et al. Oxidative stress and normal pregnancy. Clin Endocrinol (Oxf) 2002;57(5):609–13.

42. Institute of Medicine (US) Panel on micronutrients. Dietary reference intakes for vitamin A, vitamin K, arsenic, boron, chromium, copper, iodine, iron, manganese, molybdenum, nickel, silicon, vanadium, and zinc. Washington (DC): National Academies Press (US); 2001. Available at: http://www.ncbi.nlm.nih.gov/books/NBK222310/. Accessed November 12, 2018.

43. Hajhoseini L. Importance of optimal fiber consumption during pregnancy. Int J Womens Health Reprod Sci 2013;1(3):76–9.

44. Hoy MK, Goldman JD. Fiber intake of the U.S. population: what we eat in America, NHANES 2009- 2010. Food Surv Res Group Diet Data Brief 2014;(12):6.

45. Miki T, Eguchi M, Kurotani K, et al. Dietary fiber intake and depressive symptoms in Japanese employees: The Furukawa Nutrition and Health Study. Nutrition 2016;32(5):584–9.

46. Seo Y, Je Y. A comparative study of dietary habits and nutritional intakes among Korean adults according to current depression status. Asia Pac Psychiatry 2018;10(3):e12321.

47. Koh A, De Vadder F, Kovatcheva-Datchary P, et al. From dietary fiber to host physiology: short-chain fatty acids as key bacterial metabolites. Cell 2016; 165(6):1332–45.

48. Louis P, Hold GL, Flint HJ. The gut microbiota, bacterial metabolites and colorectal cancer. Nat Rev Microbiol 2014;12(10):661–72.

49. Maslowski KM, Mackay CR. Diet, gut microbiota and immune responses. Nat Immunol 2011;12(1):5–9.

50. Sun J, Wang F, Hong G, et al. Antidepressant-like effects of sodium butyrate and its possible mechanisms of action in mice exposed to chronic unpredictable mild stress. Neurosci Lett 2016;618:159–66.

51. Kelly JR, Borre Y, O' Brien C, et al. Transferring the blues: depression-associated gut microbiota induces neurobehavioural changes in the rat. J Psychiatr Res 2016;82:109–18.

52. Needell JC, Ir D, Robertson CE, et al. Maternal treatment with short-chain fatty acids modulates the intestinal microbiota and immunity and ameliorates type 1 diabetes in the offspring. PLoS One 2017;12(9):e0183786.

53. Nebholz CL, Durke KT, Yang Q, et al. Dietary fat impacts fetal growth and metabolism: uptake of chylomicron remnant core lipids by the placenta. Am J Physiol Endocrinol Metab 2011;301(2):E416–25.

54. Kim H, Kang S, Jung B-M, et al. Breast milk fatty acid composition and fatty acid intake of lactating mothers in South Korea. Br J Nutr 2017;117(04):556–61.
55. Sharma S, Fulton S. Diet-induced obesity promotes depressive-like behaviour that is associated with neural adaptations in brain reward circuitry. Int J Obes 2013;37(3):382–9.
56. Singh M. Mood, food, and obesity. Front Psychol 2014;5. https://doi.org/10.3389/fpsyg.2014.00925.
57. Cani PD, Amar J, Iglesias MA, et al. Metabolic endotoxemia initiates obesity and insulin resistance. Diabetes 2007;56(7):1761–72.
58. Devkota S, Wang Y, Musch MW, et al. Dietary-fat-induced taurocholic acid promotes pathobiont expansion and colitis in Il10 −/− mice. Nature 2012; 487(7405):104–8.
59. Ridlon JM, Harris SC, Bhowmik S, et al. Consequences of bile salt biotransformations by intestinal bacteria. Gut Microbes 2016;7(1):22–39.
60. Caesar R, Tremaroli V, Kovatcheva-Datchary P, et al. Crosstalk between gut microbiota and dietary lipids aggravates WAT inflammation through TLR signaling. Cell Metab 2015;22(4):658–68.
61. Schneeberger M, Everard A, Gómez-Valadés AG, et al. *Akkermansia muciniphila* inversely correlates with the onset of inflammation, altered adipose tissue metabolism and metabolic disorders during obesity in mice. Sci Rep 2015;5(1). https://doi.org/10.1038/srep16643.
62. Wong M-L, Inserra A, Lewis MD, et al. Inflammasome signaling affects anxiety- and depressive-like behavior and gut microbiome composition. Mol Psychiatry 2016;21(6):797–805.
63. Gohir W, Whelan FJ, Surette MG, et al. Pregnancy-related changes in the maternal gut microbiota are dependent upon the mother's periconceptional diet. Gut Microbes 2015;6(5):310–20.
64. Bodnar LM, Wisner KL. Nutrition and depression: implications for improving mental health among childbearing-aged women. Biol Psychiatry 2005;58(9): 679–85.
65. Hibbeln JR, Salem N. Dietary polyunsaturated fatty acids and depression: when cholesterol does not satisfy. Am J Clin Nutr 1995;62(1):1–9.
66. Witte AV, Kerti L, Hermannstädter HM, et al. Long-chain omega-3 fatty acids improve brain function and structure in older adults. Cereb Cortex 2014; 24(11):3059–68.
67. Larqué E, Gil-Sánchez A, Prieto-Sánchez MT, et al. Omega 3 fatty acids, gestation and pregnancy outcomes. Br J Nutr 2012;107(S2):S77–84.
68. Trujillo J, Vieira MC, Lepsch J, et al. A systematic review of the associations between maternal nutritional biomarkers and depression and/or anxiety during pregnancy and postpartum. J Affect Disord 2018;232:185–203.
69. Costantini L, Molinari R, Farinon B, et al. Impact of omega-3 fatty acids on the gut microbiota. Int J Mol Sci 2017;18(12). https://doi.org/10.3390/ijms18122645.
70. Stephens TV, Payne M, Ball RO, et al. Protein requirements of healthy pregnant women during early and late gestation are higher than current recommendations. J Nutr 2015;145(1):73–8.
71. The role of protein and amino acids in sustaining and enhancing performance. Washington, DC: National Academies Press; 1999. https://doi.org/10.17226/9620.
72. Laterra J, Keep R, Betz LA, et al. Blood-brain-cerebrospinal fluid barriers. In: Siegel GJ, editor. Basic neurochemistry: molecular, cellular and medical aspects. 5th edition. New York: Raven Press; 1994. p. 681–98.

73. Byerley LO, Samuelson D, Blanchard E, et al. Changes in the gut microbial communities following addition of walnuts to the diet. J Nutr Biochem 2017;48: 94–102.

74. Young SN. Behavioral effects of dietary neurotransmitter precursors: basic and clinical aspects. Neurosci Biobehav Rev 1996;20(2):313–23.

75. Ogawa S, Fujii T, Koga N, et al. Plasma L-tryptophan concentration in major depressive disorder: new data and meta-analysis. J Clin Psychiatry 2014; 75(09):e906–15.

76. Badawy AA-B. Tryptophan metabolism, disposition and utilization in pregnancy. Biosci Rep 2015;35(5):e00261.

77. Russell WR, Duncan SH, Scobbie L, et al. Major phenylpropanoid-derived metabolites in the human gut can arise from microbial fermentation of protein. Mol Nutr Food Res 2013;57(3):523–35.

78. Valladares R, Bojilova L, Potts AH, et al. *Lactobacillus johnsonii* inhibits indole-amine 2,3-dioxygenase and alters tryptophan metabolite levels in BioBreeding rats. FASEB J 2013;27(4):1711–20.

79. Baskin R, Hill B, Jacka FN, et al. Antenatal dietary patterns and depressive symptoms during pregnancy and early post-partum: Antenatal dietary patterns and depressive symptoms. Matern Child Nutr 2017;13(1):e12218.

80. Fowles ER, Stang J, Bryant M, et al. Stress, depression, social support, and eating habits reduce diet quality in the first trimester in low-income women: a pilot study. J Acad Nutr Diet 2012;112(10):1619–25.

81. Bergmans RS, Malecki KM. The association of dietary inflammatory potential with depression and mental well-being among U.S. adults. Prev Med 2017;99: 313–9.

82. Sánchez-Villegas A, Delgado-Rodríguez M, Alonso A, et al. Association of the mediterranean dietary pattern with the incidence of depression: the Seguimiento Universidad de Navarra/University of Navarra follow-up (SUN) cohort. Arch Gen Psychiatry 2009;66(10):1090.

83. Rienks J, Dobson AJ, Mishra GD. Mediterranean dietary pattern and prevalence and incidence of depressive symptoms in mid-aged women: results from a large community-based prospective study. Eur J Clin Nutr 2013;67(1):75–82.

84. Jacka FN, O'Neil A, Opie R, et al. A randomised controlled trial of dietary improvement for adults with major depression (the 'SMILES' trial). BMC Med 2017;15(1). https://doi.org/10.1186/s12916-017-0791-y.

85. Sánchez-Villegas A, Martínez-González MA, Estruch R, et al. Mediterranean dietary pattern and depression: the PREDIMED randomized trial. BMC Med 2013; 11(1). https://doi.org/10.1186/1741-7015-11-208.

86. Sandhu KV, Sherwin E, Schellekens H, et al. Feeding the microbiota-gut-brain axis: diet, microbiome, and neuropsychiatry. Transl Res 2017;179:223–44.

87. Bruce-Keller AJ, Salbaum JM, Luo M, et al. Obese-type gut microbiota induce neurobehavioral changes in the absence of obesity. Biol Psychiatry 2015; 77(7):607–15.

88. Garcia-Mantrana I, Selma-Royo M, Alcantara C, et al. Shifts on gut microbiota associated to mediterranean diet adherence and specific dietary intakes on general adult population. Front Microbiol 2018;9. https://doi.org/10.3389/fmicb.2018.00890.

89. Nava GM, Carbonero F, Ou J, et al. Hydrogenotrophic microbiota distinguish native Africans from African and European Americans: diet and colonic hydrogenotrophs. Environ Microbiol Rep 2012;4(3):307–15.

90. Neyrinck AM, Possemiers S, Verstraete W, et al. Dietary modulation of clostridial cluster XIVa gut bacteria (*Roseburia* spp.) by chitin–glucan fiber improves host metabolic alterations induced by high-fat diet in mice. J Nutr Biochem 2012; 23(1):51–9.
91. Jiang H, Ling Z, Zhang Y, et al. Altered fecal microbiota composition in patients with major depressive disorder. Brain Behav Immun 2015;48:186–94.
92. Pendyala S, Walker JM, Holt PR. A high-fat diet is associated with endotoxemia that originates from the gut. Gastroenterology 2012;142(5):1100–1.e2.
93. Haro C, Montes-Borrego M, Rangel-Zúñiga OA, et al. Two healthy diets modulate gut microbial community improving insulin sensitivity in a human obese population. J Clin Endocrinol Metab 2016;101(1):233–42.
94. Dai J, Jones DP, Goldberg J, et al. Association between adherence to the Mediterranean diet and oxidative stress. Am J Clin Nutr 2008;88(5):1364–70.
95. Cox EQ, Sowa NA, Meltzer-Brody SE, et al. The perinatal depression treatment cascade: Baby steps toward improving outcomes. J Clin Psychiatry 2016;1189–200. https://doi.org/10.4088/JCP.15r10174.
96. DiGiulio DB, Callahan BJ, McMurdie PJ, et al. Temporal and spatial variation of the human microbiota during pregnancy. Proc Natl Acad Sci U S A 2015; 112(35):11060–5.
97. Zeevi D, Korem T, Zmora N, et al. Personalized nutrition by prediction of glycemic responses. Cell 2015;163(5):1079–94.
98. Slykerman RF, Hood F, Wickens K, et al. Effect of *Lactobacillus rhamnosus* HN001 in pregnancy on postpartum symptoms of depression and anxiety: a randomised double-blind placebo-controlled trial. EBioMedicine 2017;24: 159–65.
99. Macedo D, Filho AJMC, Soares de Sousa CN, et al. Antidepressants, antimicrobials or both? Gut microbiota dysbiosis in depression and possible implications of the antimicrobial effects of antidepressant drugs for antidepressant effectiveness. J Affect Disord 2017;208:22–32.
100. Karine de Sousa A, Rocha JE, Gonçalves de Souza T, et al. New roles of fluoxetine in pharmacology: antibacterial effect and modulation of antibiotic activity. Microb Pathog 2018;123:368–71.

The Microbiota and Pancreatic Cancer

Tomasz M. Karpiński, MSc Biol, DDS, MD, PhD, DSc

KEYWORDS

- Pancreatic cancer • Microbiota • Carcinogenesis • Chronic inflammation
- Antiapoptotic activity • Helicobacter pylori • Porphyromonas gingivalis • HBV

KEY POINTS

- *Helicobacter pylori*, oral periopathogens (eg, Porphyromonas, Fusobacterium, Aggregatibacter, Prevotella, or Capnocytophaga), and hepatitis B (HBV) and C viruses (HCV) can affect the development of pancreatic cancer.
- Main mechanisms of action of carcinogenic microbiota depend on the development of chronic inflammation and antiapoptotic activity.
- Distant infections (eg, gastric ulcer, gingivitis, periodontitis) can lead to translocation of bacteria to the pancreas and the beginning of the cancer process.
- Infections of HBV or HCV are essential risk factors not only for liver cancer but also for pancreatic cancer.

INTRODUCTION

Pancreatic cancer belongs to the most aggressive and lethal diseases. The prognosis for this cancer is weak, and the 5-year survival rate is less than 7%. The most common histologic type is pancreatic ductal adenocarcinoma.[1] In 2015 approximately 367,000 new cases of pancreatic cancer were diagnosed worldwide.[2] The number of patients with pancreatic cancer increases dramatically, and in 2018 there were 458,918 new cases and 432,242 deaths. It means that as many as 94% of patients with this disease die. Because of its poor prognosis, pancreatic cancer is the seventh leading cause of cancer death.[3] In the general worldwide population, the incidence is 8 cases per 100,000 person years and mortality is seven deaths per 100,000 person years.[4] In the United States, cancer of the pancreas is the fourth leading cause of cancer mortality in humans.[1] It is predicted that by 2030 the number of pancreatic cancers will increase twice in the United States.[5]

Data suggest that the progression of pancreatic cancer from preinvasive changes to invasive disease arises from the gradual accumulation of gene mutations. The most

Disclosure Statement: The author has nothing to disclose.
Department of Medical Microbiology, Poznań University of Medical Sciences, Wieniawskiego 3, Poznań 61-712, Poland
E-mail addresses: tkarpin@ump.edu.pl; tkarpin@interia.pl

important in pancreatic ductal adenocarcinoma include the activation of KRAS onco-gene (Kirsten rat sarcoma viral oncogene homolog) and inactivation of the following genes: tumor suppressor gene p16/CDKN2A (p16/cyclin-dependent kinase inhibitor 2 A), tumor suppressor gene TP53 (tumor protein p53), and SMAD4 gene (SMAD family member 4).[6–8] Mutations of the abovementioned genes are observed in more than 50% of the cancers. KRAS oncogene is activated in 95% of invasive ductal adenocarcinomas, whereas the p16/CDKN2A gene is inactivated in about 95% and the TP53 in 75% of pancreatic cancers.[9] Mutations in SMAD4 gene are associated with poor prognosis and metastases.[10]

Many factors are affecting the development of pancreatic cancer. The most important risk factor is smoking.[11] Smokers have 2.2-fold higher risk of pancreatic cancer compared with nonsmokers.[12] A second risk factor is alcohol consumption, which increases the hazard of pancreatic cancer by 60%.[13,14] Other risk factors are type 2 diabetes mellitus and obesity.[15,16] In patients with type 2 diabetes mellitus a moderate intestinal dysbiosis occur, characterized by a decrease in butyrate-producing *Roseburia intestinalis* and *Faecalibacterium prausnitzii*.[17] Intestinal microbiota may play an essential role in the pathogenesis of diabetes mellitus by influencing body weight, bile acid metabolism, proinflammatory activity, insulin resistance, and modulation of gut hormones.[18] Obesity leads, among others, to increased production of adipokines (among others leptin, tumor necrosis factor alpha [TNF-α], interleukin 6 [IL-6]) that affect the severity of inflammation, the increase of insulin resistance, and changes in intestinal microbiota.[19] Obesity may exacerbate acute pancreatitis by damaging the intestinal mucosal barrier. Studies on rats presented that pancreatic pathologic score, intestinal permeability, and serum leptin were significantly higher in obese rats with acute pancreatitis (AP) than in nonobese rats with AP. Moreover, in obese rats with AP the dysbiosis of intestinal microbiota was detected.[20] In addition, it was shown that high body mass index could reduce response to chemotherapy.[21] Inflammation plays a crucial role in pancreatic cancer.[22] Smoking and obesity have an impact on increasing the risk of pancreatic cancer by causing systemic inflammation. In patients with chronic pancreatitis an increased probability of pancreatic cancer has been observed.[23,24] Some studies have shown positive associations of poor oral health, periodontitis, and tooth loss with an increased risk of pancreatic cancer development.[25–28] Gingivitis and periodontitis are also associated with an excess risk of pancreatic cancer mortality.[25,29]

Molecular studies, especially next-generation sequencing, revealed that changes in microbiota are essential for the development of oral, colorectal, and pancreatic cancers. *H. pylori* and oral bacteria belonging to periopathogens, *Porphyromonas gingivalis* and *Fusobacterium nucleatum,* seem to have particular importance in colorectal and pancreatic cancers.[30–35] In cancer changes have been demonstrated also other bacteria, among others from genera *Bacteroides, Leptotrichia, Streptococcus, Capnocytophaga, Prevotella, Neisseria, and Veillonella.*[36–42]

In this review bacteria and viruses oncogenic for the pancreatic tissues are presented. Possible mechanisms of carcinogenic action of microorganisms are also described (**Fig. 1**).

CARCINOGENIC BACTERIA

Some studies demonstrated a link between significant periodontal pathogen *P. gingivalis* and pancreatic cancer. Michaud and colleagues[17] studied antibodies against 25 oral bacteria in a prospective cohort. In patients with pancreatic ductal cancer, levels of antibodies against periodontal pathogen *P gingivalis* ATTC 53978 were significantly

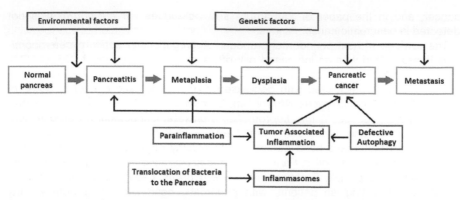

Fig. 1. Overview of pancreatic cancer development and related risk factors. (*Data from* Refs.[32,61,145])

higher than in controls. High amounts of *P gingivalis* were associated with a 2-fold increase in pancreatic cancer risk (odds ratio [OR] = 2.14). Simultaneously, high levels of antibodies against nonpathogenic oral bacteria were linked to a lower risk of pancreatic cancer. In the second cohort study, a higher risk of pancreatic cancer was associated with carriage of *P gingivalis* (OR = 1.60). This association was observed both for low carriers and high carriers.[34] It was demonstrated that *P gingivalis* is associated with increased orodigestive cancer mortality, including pancreatic cancer. Pancreatic cancer mortality is also associated with periodontitis, and mortality risk increased with increasing severity of periodontal disease. Increased cancer mortality was observed in patients with greater levels of serum immunoglobulin G against *P gingivalis*. The investigators suggested that *P gingivalis* is a biomarker for risk of death due to colorectal and pancreatic cancers[29] (**Fig. 2**).

Other periodontal bacteria belonging to *Fusobacterium* species were detected in 8.8% of the pancreatic cancer tissue specimens. *Fusobacterium* species were discovered mainly in pancreatic tail cancer (22%) and to a lesser extent in the head (7.9%) or body cancer (8.0%). In *Fusobacterium*-positive cases significantly higher mortality rates and shorter survival were also observed.[33] Contrary, in studies of Fan and colleagues[34] *Fusobacteria* were associated with decreased risk of pancreatic ductal

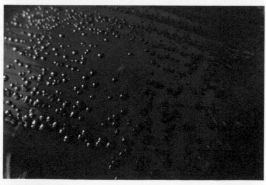

Fig. 2. The culture of *Porphyromonas gingivalis* (black-pigmented colonies) on the Columbia agar with sheep blood.

cancer, and in the paper of Yamamura and colleagues[44] F nucleatum was not detected in pancreatic cancer tissues.

The carriage of next periodontal pathogen Aggregatibacter actinomycetemcomitans is associated with an increased risk of pancreatic ductal cancer (OR = 2.20). Simultaneously, carriage of Tannerella forsythia, Prevotella intermedia, and genus Leptotrichia was associated with decreased risk of pancreatic cancer.[34] Some of the oral bacteria (Actinomyces, Atopobium, Campylobacter, Catonella, Corynebacterium, Filifactor, Fusobacterium, Leptotrichia, Moraxella, Oribacterium, Peptostreptococcus, Rothia, and Tannerella) were overrepresented in the tongue coating of patients with pancreatic head carcinoma. In healthy controls, the tongue coating was enriched in Haemophilus, Paraprevotella, and Porphyromonas. The investigators suggested that especially Fusobacterium, Haemophilus, Leptotrichia, and Porphyromonas could distinguish patients with pancreatic head carcinoma from healthy persons.[41]

In studies of Olson and colleagues,[45] higher levels of Streptococcus thermophilus were found in pancreatic ductal adenocarcinoma cases compared with controls. In controls higher levels of Haemophilus parainfluenzae and Neisseria flaviscens were found. In the research of Del Castillo and colleagues,[42] Fusobacterium, Porphyromonas, Pyramidobacter, Capnocytophaga, Prevotella, Selenomonas, and Gemella were present in higher mean relative abundance in subjects with pancreatic cancer than in persons without cancer. Simultaneously, taxa more common in pancreatic cancer were Haemophilus, Pyramidobacter, Aggregatibacter, Prevotella, and Gemella. In almost all noncancer tissue samples Lactobacillus taxa were present.

According to Torres and colleagues,[40] patients with pancreatic ductal cancer had significantly higher levels of Leptotrichia and lower levels of P gingivalis in the saliva. They also had a higher relative abundance of Bacteroides and lower relative abundances of Neisseria elongata and A actinomycetemcomitans, although these results were not significant. In the paper of Lin and colleagues,[39] in patients with pancreatitis and with pancreatic cancer compared with the control group Bacteroides genus was significantly more abundant. In addition, Corynebacterium and Aggregatibacter were less abundant in pancreatic cancer and pancreatitis groups compared with controls. Farrell and colleagues in their study[38] described differences in the microflora of pancreatic ductal cancer compared with healthy participants, specifically Streptococcus, Prevotella, Campylobacter, Granulicatella, Atopobium, and Neisseria. In patients with pancreatic ductal cancer, N elongata and Streptococcus mitis were found to be significantly lower, whereas Granulicatella adiacens was higher compared with healthy participants. The investigators concluded that the combination of N elongata and S mitis biomarkers yielded 96.4% sensitivity and 82.1% specificity in distinguishing patients with pancreatic cancer from healthy subjects. Similarly, decreased level of antibodies against S mitis in patients with pancreatic ductal cancer was observed by Michaud and colleagues.[43] Half and colleagues[46] found the 2-fold higher concentration of Bacteroides, Verrucomicrobia, Sutterella, Veillonella, Bacteroides, Odoribacter and Akkermansia in patients with pancreatic ductal cancer compared with controls. Two groups of bacteria, Firmicutes and Actinobacteria, were lower in pancreatic cancer compared with controls.

Some bacteria, for example, Enterococcus and Enterobacter, can survive in pancreatic juice and bile. Enterococcus faecalis was detected frequently in pancreatic tissue from patients with chronic pancreatitis and pancreatic cancer. Moreover, the titers of antibodies against E faecalis capsular polysaccharide were increased in chronic pancreatitis and pancreatic cancer compared with healthy donors and patients with colorectal cancer.[47]

Helicobacter pylori are the most well-known carcinogenic bacteria. It is a class I carcinogen associated with the development of peptic ulcer disease and chronic gastritis. In some patients, *H pylori* lead to the development of gastric adenocarcinoma and gastric mucosa–associated lymphoid tissue lymphoma.[48,49] The prospective cohort study reported that persons with *H pylori* antibodies or CagA positive *H pylori* strains had increased risk of developing pancreatic cancer (OR = 1.87 and OR = 2.01, respectively).[37] In the pancreas, *Helicobacter* DNA was detected in tumor tissues. DNA was confirmed in 75% of patients with exocrine cancer, 57% with neuroendocrine cancer, 38% with multiple endocrine neoplasia, and 60% with chronic pancreatitis. *Helicobacter* DNA was not detected in benign pancreatic diseases and normal pancreas.[50] A positive association between *H pylori* infection and pancreatic cancer was also presented by Raderer and colleagues.[36] They showed that 65% of patients with pancreatic cancer were found to be seropositive to *H pylori*. Some systematic review and meta-analyses found that *H pylori*-positive patients had a significantly higher risk of developing pancreatic cancer. Significant correlation between *H pylori* infection and pancreatic cancer was presented by Guo and colleagues[51] (OR = 1.45), Xiao and colleagues[52] (OR = 1.47), and Trikudanathan and colleagues[53] (OR = 1.38). However, a case-control study from Poland reported no dependence between seropositivity of *H pylori* (OR = 1.27) or CagA (OR = 0.90) and risk of pancreatic cancer.[54] Similar results were presented in meta-analyses of Liu and colleagues[55] (OR = 1.09), Schulte and colleagues[56] (OR = 1.00), and Wang and colleagues[57] (OR = 1.06). Interesting results were obtained by Chen and colleagues,[58] which did not detect a relationship between pancreatic cancer and *H pylori* infection (OR = 0.99) but observed that CagA-negative *H pylori* strains may be a potential risk factor of pancreatic cancer (OR = 1.47).

CARCINOGENIC MECHANISMS OF ACTION OF BACTERIA

Oral pathogens, for example, *Porphyromonas*, *Prevotella*, and *Fusobacterium*, can cause chronic inflammation both in the oral cavity and in the gastrointestinal tract. Bacteria lead to the production of inflammatory mediators, including IL-1β, IL-6, TNF-α, and matrix metalloproteinases (MMPs).[59] IL-1β and TNF-α are produced in response to bacterial lipopolysaccharide (LPS). LPS can activate toll-like receptor 4 (TLR4) on immune cells in the tumor microenvironment. It leads to activation of the nuclear factor-κB (NF-κB) and mitogen-activated protein kinase (MAPK) signaling pathways in immune cells and promotes pancreatic tumor development.[60] TLR4 also induce expression of NACHT, LRR, and PYD domains containing protein 3 (NLRP3) inflammasome. The NLRP3 inflammasome affects releasing of IL-1β and IL-18.[61] IL-1β stimulates the release of prostaglandins, proinflammatory IL-6, TNF-α, and MMPs, among others.[62,63] This cytokine activates endothelial cells to produce proangiogenic factors and is associated with angiogenesis, tumor progression, and invasiveness.[64,65] The tumor invasion by local extracellular matrix degradation affects MMP-9 induced by IL-1β.[66] The increasing of the MMP expression also leads to IL-6. This cytokine additionally induces oxidative stress, leads to mitochondrial damage,[67,68] and is involved in the progression of cell cycle and suppression of apoptosis.[69] In the pancreatic cancer group as compared with healthy controls statistically significant higher levels of C-reactive protein and IL-6 were stated.[70] TNF-α induces production of reactive oxygen compounds, leukotrienes, prostaglandins, and MMPs.[71] Low doses of TNF-α are related to tumor promotion by activation of oncogenic Wnt and NF-κB signaling pathways.[72,73] Experimental evidence in a mouse model of pancreatic cancer suggests that lipopolysaccharide can activate TLR4 on immune cells in the tumor microenvironment and promote pancreatic tumor development through activation of the NF-κB and MAPK signaling pathways in immune cells.[60] Induction of MMPs and angiogenic factors by TNF-α affects cell motility and tumor invasion.[74,75] During an inflammatory response, TNF-α, IL-6, and TGF-β affect the epithelial and immune cells, which are starting to produce reactive oxygen species (ROS) and reactive nitrogen species (RNS).[76,77] Some species of *Streptococcus* (eg, *S mitis*), in the oral cavity involved in this process, produce hydrogen peroxide (H_2O_2).[78] *E faecalis* produces extracellular superoxide and derivative oxygen species, which can lead to DNA mutations in host cells.[79]

P gingivalis also acts antiapoptotic by activation of Jak1/Akt/Stat3 signaling,[80,81] activation of cyclin/cyclin-dependent kinase (CDK), and inhibition of the p53 tumor suppressor.[82] *P gingivalis* inactivates proapoptotic Bcl-2–associated death promoter, simultaneously inhibiting caspase-9[83] and activating the antiapoptotic Bcl-2.[84] *P gingivalis* also produces gingipains, which are cysteine proteinases, and activate MMP-9, which promote carcinoma cell migration and invasion.[85] *P gingivalis* together with *P intermedia, T forsythia,* and *Treponema denticola* produce peptidylarginine deiminase (PAD) enzyme. PAD can be responsible for p53 mutation, which is a risk factor in pancreatic cancer.[86,87] *P gingivalis* can additionally modulate ROS, leading to inflammation and cancer development[88] (**Fig. 3**).

F nucleatum LPS activated inflammatory cytokines such as IL-1β, IL-6, and TNF-α. The chronic inflammatory process leads to loss of periodontal attachment and tissue damage.[89] *F nucleatum* infection modulates several antiapoptotic pathways. Bacterium induces NF-κB signaling as a consequence of the TLR activation.[90] *F nucleatum* promotes carcinogenesis by modulating E-cadherin/β-catenin signaling via its FadA adhesin/invasin. Numerous changes occur, such as the increase of transcriptional activity of Wnt, activation of proinflammatory cytokines and oncogenes, and stimulation

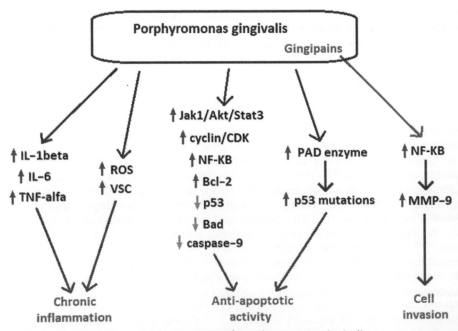

Fig. 3. Mechanisms of carcinogenic activity of *Porphyromonas gingivalis*.

of cancer cell proliferation.[91] FadA is a crucial virulence factor of *F nucleatum*. This protein changes macrophage infiltration and methylation of the CDKN2A promoter in cancer areas.[92] LPS of *F nucleatum* activates β-catenin signaling. In this process an enhancement of the expression of β-catenin, oncogenes C-myc, and cyclin D1 is observed.[93,94] In addition, *F nucleatum* activates p38 and has an impact on the secretion of MMP-9 and MMP-13. These metalloproteinases play a critical role in the invasion of cancer cells and metastasis[95] (**Fig. 4**).

Some periodontal pathogens, for example, *A actinomycetemcomitans*, *F nucleatum*, *P gingivalis*, and *P intermedia* produce volatile sulfur compounds (VSCs). To VSCs belong hydrogen sulfide, mercaptans, dimethyl sulfide, and dimethyl disulfide, among others. All these compounds play a role in the periodontitis supporting chronic inflammation.[96,97] Hydrogen sulfide is a known genotoxic agent and coworks with cystathionine-β-synthase. Both affect tumor cell proliferation and migration and enhance tumor angiogenesis.[98,99] Hooper and colleagues[100] presented in oral squamous cell carcinoma saccharolytic and aciduric streptococci. *Streptococcus* sp. produce acids, including lactic acid,[101] which change tumor microenvironment to acidic and hypoxic.[102,103] Streptococci such as *Streptococcus gordonii*, *S mitis*, *Streptococcus oralis*, *Streptococcus salivarius*, and *Streptococcus sanguinis* possess the enzyme alcohol dehydrogenase (ADH), which metabolizes alcohol to carcinogenic acetaldehyde.[104,105] Extremely high ADH activity was observed in genus *Neisseria*, which can play an essential role in alcohol-related carcinogenesis in humans.[106]

H pylori contain cytotoxin-associated gene A (CagA) and secret virulence factors, such as vacuolating cytotoxin A (VacA) and urease. These factors contribute to carcinogenesis by the promotion of chronic inflammation, oxidative stress, and host DNA damage.[107,108] CagA protein can affect the shape, motility, and proliferation of the cells. The presence of CagA in a strain results in an increased risk of gastric

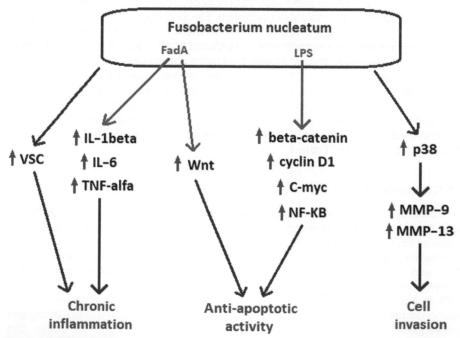

Fig. 4. Mechanisms of carcinogenic activity of *Fusobacterium nucleatum*.

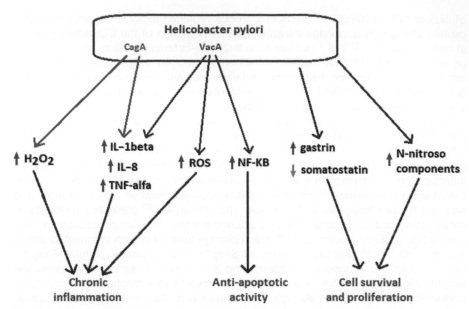

Fig. 5. Mechanisms of carcinogenic activity of *Helicobacter pylori*.

carcinogenesis. CagA also increases TNF-α, IL-8, and hydrogen peroxide levels and oxidative DNA damage leading to cause double-strand breaks of DNA.[109–112] Upregulation of IL-1β, IL-8, and COX-2 in patients with chronic gastritis has a crucial clinical implication in gastric carcinogenesis.[113] VacA is a toxin-inducing inflammatory cytokine after entering the cells. It affects the production of ROS and activation of NF-κB.[114] Effect of *H pylori* on pancreatic cancer is probably associated with increased gastrin and decreased somatostatin secretion. Elevated gastrin levels could stimulate pancreatic cell growth and proliferation. Simultaneously, gastrin increases the susceptibility of the pancreas to carcinogens. Reduced levels of somatostatin could allow for increased pancreatic cancer growth.[37] *H pylori* activity also increases the formation of N-nitroso components, which can initiate the carcinogenesis process.[115] Probably, *H pylori* growth in the gastric corpus mucosa leads to hypochlorhydria and bacterial overgrowth. The increased amount of bacteria results in accelerated production of endogenous carcinogens N-nitrosamines, which are transported to the host pancreas via bloodstream[116,117] (**Fig. 5**). Bacterial species implicated in pancreatic cancer are presented in **Table 1**.

CARCINOGENIC VIRUSES

Some studies confirm that hepatitis B (HBV) and hepatitis C viruses (HCV) are linked with pancreatic cancer development. Jin and colleagues[118] revealed that the prevalence of HBV DNA and anti-HBc were significantly increased in patients with pancreatic cancer compared with healthy controls (OR = 1.87 and OR = 1.91, respectively). Ben and colleagues[119] reported that chronic and inactive HBV surface antigen (HBsAg) carrier state leads to the significantly increased risk of pancreatic cancer (OR = 1.60). The dependence between HBV infection and pancreatic cancer was demonstrated in the meta-analyses of Li and colleagues[120] (OR = 1.403), Wang and colleagues[121] (OR = 1.60 and 1.76), Luo and colleagues[122] (RR = 3.83), and Majumder and colleagues[123] (OR = 1.50). In the meta-analysis conducted by Xing

Table 1
Changes in an amount of bacterial species implicated in pancreatic cancer

No.	Microbial Alterations—Increases	Microbial Alterations—Decreases	References
1.	*Helicobacter pylori*		36,37,50–53
2.	*Porphyromonas gingivalis*		29,34,41–43
3.	*Fusobacterium* sp.		33,41,42
4.	*Bacteroides* sp.		39,40,46
5.	*Leptotrichia* sp.		40,41
6.	*Aggregatibacter actinomycetemcomitans*		34
7.	*Akkermansia* sp.		46
8.	*Capnocytophaga* sp.		42
9.	*Enterococcus faecalis*		47
10.	*Gemella* sp.		42
11.	*Granulicatella adiacens*		38
12.	*Haemophilus* sp.		41
13.	*Odoribacter* sp.		46
14.	*Prevotella* sp.		42
15.	*Pyramidobacter* sp.		42
16.	*Selenomonas* sp.		42
17.	*Streptococcus thermophilus*		45
18.	*Sutterella* sp.		46
19.	*Veillonella* sp.		46
20.	*Verrucomicrobia* sp.		46
21.		*Streptococcus mitis*	38,43
22.		*Aggregatibacter* sp.	39
23.		*Corynebacterium* sp.	39
24.		*Fusobacterium* sp.	34
25.		*Haemophilus parainfluenzae*	45
26.		*Leptotrichia* sp.	34
27.		*Neisseria elongata*	38
28.		*Neisseria flavescens*	45
29.		*Prevotella intermedia*	34
30.		*P gingivalis*	40
31.		*Tannerella forsythia*	34

and colleagues,[124] they confirm that HBV infection is associated with an increased risk of pancreatic cancer in HBsAg-positive patients (OR = 1.28). Luo and colleagues[122] in the meta-analysis showed that the pancreatic cancer risk was positively correlated with HBV infection (risk ratio [RR] = 1.39 in chronic HBV carriers, 1.41 in past exposure to HBV, and 3.83 in active HBV infection). Contrary, there are also papers in which investigators found no association between HBV infection and pancreatic cancer. Andersen and colleagues[125] presented that the incidence rate ratio for pancreatic cancer among HBV-infected patients was 0.9. In another study the investigators did not observe a statistically significant association between the anti-HBc presence and the risk of pancreatic cancer (hazard ratio [HR] = 1.22).[126]

Huang and colleagues[127] indicated that HCV infection might be associated with an increased risk of pancreatic cancer (standardized incidence ratio = 2.1). In the paper of Xing and colleagues[124] they confirm that HCV infections can increase the risk of pancreatic cancer in anti-HCV-positive patients (OR = 1.21). In the JPHC study, the investigators did not observe a statistically significant association between the anti-HCV presence and the risk of pancreatic cancer (HR = 0.69).[126] Also, Fiorino and colleagues[128] observed no relationship between anti-HCV positivity and pancreatic adenocarcinoma risk (RR = 1.16).

CARCINOGENIC MECHANISMS OF ACTION OF VIRUSES

In HBV and HCV infections activation of oncogenes and high level of mutations, including TP53 and CTNNB1 genes, were demonstrated. Somatic mutations were also detected in genes that occurred in oncogenic pathways, including telomere maintenance, Wnt signaling, p53/cell cycle, oxidative stress, epigenetic regulator, JAK/STAT, and others.[129,130] Both viruses lead additionally to the generation of ROS and RNS.[131] Both pathogens might replicate in the pancreas and induce chronic inflammation and injury in this organ. Chronic damage of pancreas may cause the development of metaplasia in tissues.[132] In HBV the HBx gene is primarily related to hepatocarcinogenesis. HBx is a known transcription activator through its interaction among others with epidermal growth factor receptor, c-myc, c-jun, c-fos, TP53, AP-1, NF-κB, and SP1.[133–136] HBx can affect cellular proliferation[137] and inhibit p53-mediated apoptosis.[138] The PreS2 transcription activators can activate transcription factors AP-1 and NF-κB leading to cell proliferation.[139] In HCV the core protein is involved in cell signaling, transcription activation, apoptosis, and transformation. The core protein induces reactive oxygen species and implicates in cellular proliferation, cell cycle control, and tumor formation by binding to p53 and pRb tumor suppressor proteins.[140–142] The E2 protein can inhibit T and NK cells, thereby promoting cell survival and proliferation. The NS3 protein can interact with p21 and p53 proteins,[143] whereas NS5A protein can lead to the suppression of the host immune response and inhibition of apoptosis[144] (**Fig. 6**).

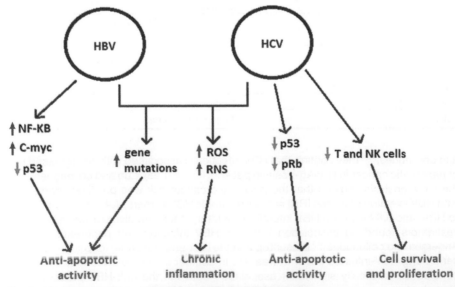

Fig. 6. Mechanisms of carcinogenic activities of HBV and HCV.

SUMMARY

Research indicates that bacteria and viruses can be essential carcinogenic agents. It has been shown that mainly *H pylori* and oral periopathogens *P gingivalis*, *Fusobacterium* sp., *Aggregatibacter* sp., *Prevotella* sp., or *Capnocytophaga* sp have a role in the development of pancreatic cancer. These microorganisms lead to chronic inflammation, antiapoptotic changes, cell survival, and cell invasion. Among viruses, infections of HBV or HCV are essential risk factors not only for liver cancer but also for pancreatic cancer.

REFERENCES

1. Siegel RL, Miller KD, Jemal A. Cancer statistics. 2017. CA Cancer J Clin 2017; 67:7–30.
2. Kleeff J, Korc M, Apte M, et al. Pancreatic cancer. Nat Rev Dis Primers 2016;2: 16022.
3. Bray F, Ferlay J, Soerjomataram I, et al. Global cancer statistics 2018: GLOBO-CAN estimates of incidence and mortality worldwide for 36 cancers in 185 countries. CA Cancer J Clin 2018;68(6):394–424.
4. Xiao AY, Tan MLY, Wu LM, et al. Global incidence and mortality of pancreatic diseases: a systematic review, meta-analysis, and meta-regression of population-based cohort studies. Lancet Gastroenterol Hepatol 2016;1:45–55.
5. Rahib L, Smith BD, Aizenberg R, et al. Projecting cancer incidence and deaths to 2030: the unexpected burden of thyroid, liver, and pancreas cancers in the United States. Cancer Res 2014;74(11):2913–21.
6. Hruban RH, Maitra A, Goggins M. Update on pancreatic intraepithelial neoplasia. Int J Clin Exp Pathol 2008;1:306–16.
7. Hidalgo M. Pancreatic cancer. N Engl J Med 2010;362(17):1605–17.
8. Aier I, Semwal R, Sharma A, et al. A systematic assessment of statistics, risk factors, and underlying features involved in pancreatic cancer. Cancer Epidemiol 2019;58:104–10.
9. Jones S, Zhang X, Parsons DW, et al. Core signaling pathways in human pancreatic cancers revealed by global genomic analyses. Science 2008;321: 1801–6.
10. Blackford A, Serrano OK, Wolfgang CL, et al. SMAD4 gene mutations are associated with poor prognosis in pancreatic cancer. Clin Cancer Res 2009;15: 4674–9.
11. Alexandrov LB, Ju YS, Haase K, et al. Mutational signatures associated with tobacco smoking in human cancer. Science 2016;354:618–22.
12. Goral V. Pancreatic cancer: pathogenesis and diagnosis. Asian Pac J Cancer Prev 2015;16(14):5619–24.
13. Genkinger JM, Spiegelman D, Anderson KE, et al. Alcohol intake and pancreatic cancer risk: a pooled analysis of fourteen cohort studies. Cancer Epidemiol Biomarkers Prev 2009;18:765–76.
14. Tramacere I, Scotti L, Jenab M, et al. Alcohol drinking and pancreatic cancer risk: a meta-analysis of the dose-risk relation. Int J Cancer 2010;126:1474–86.
15. Arslan AA, Helzlsouer KJ, Kooperberg C, et al. Anthropometric measures, body mass index, and pancreatic cancer: a pooled analysis from the Pancreatic Cancer Cohort Consortium (PanScan). Arch Intern Med 2010;170:791–802.
16. Pothuraju R, Rachagani S, Junker WM, et al. Pancreatic cancer associated with obesity and diabetes: an alternative approach for its targeting. J Exp Clin Cancer Res 2018;37(1):319.

17. Qin J, Li Y, Cai Z, et al. A metagenome-wide association study of gut microbiota in type 2 diabetes. Nature 2012;490:55–60.
18. Han JL, Lin HL. Intestinal microbiota and type 2 diabetes: from mechanism insights to therapeutic perspective. World J Gastroenterol 2014;20:17737–45.
19. Xu M, Jung X, Hines OJ, et al. Obesity and pancreatic cancer: overview of epidemiology and potential prevention by weight loss. Pancreas 2018;47(2):158–62.
20. Ye C, Liu L, Ma X, et al. Obesity aggravates acute pancreatitis via damaging intestinal mucosal barrier and changing microbiota composition in rats. Sci Rep 2019;9(1):69.
21. Cascetta P, Cavaliere A, Piro G, et al. Pancreatic cancer and obesity: molecular mechanisms of cell transformation and chemoresistance. Int J Mol Sci 2018;19(11):E3331.
22. Greer JB, Whitcomb DC. Inflammation and pancreatic cancer: an evidence-based review. Curr Opin Pharmacol 2009;9:411–8.
23. Talamini G, Falconi M, Bassi C, et al. Incidence of cancer in the course of chronic pancreatitis. Am J Gastroenterol 1999;94:1253–60.
24. Malka D, Hammel P, Maire F, et al. Risk of pancreatic adenocarcinoma in chronic pancreatitis. Gut 2002;51:849–52.
25. Hujoel PP, Drangsholt M, Spiekerman C, et al. An exploration of the periodontitis cancer association. Ann Epidemiol 2003;13:312–6.
26. Stolzenberg-Solomon RZ, Dodd KW, Blaser MJ, et al. Tooth loss, pancreatic cancer, and *Helicobacter pylori*. Am J Clin Nutr 2003;78:176–81.
27. Michaud DS, Joshipura K, Giovannucci E, et al. A prospective study of periodontal disease and pancreatic cancer in US male health professionals. J Natl Cancer Inst 2007;99:171–5.
28. Chang JS, Tsai CR, Chen LT, et al. Investigating the association between periodontal disease and risk of pancreatic cancer. Pancreas 2016;45(1):134–41.
29. Ahn J, Segers S, Hayes RB. Periodontal disease, *Porphyromonas gingivalis* serum antibody levels and orodigestive cancer mortality. Carcinogenesis 2012;33(5):1055–8.
30. Castellarin M, Warren RL, Freeman JD, et al. *Fusobacterium nucleatum* infection is prevalent in human colorectal carcinoma. Genome Res 2012;22(2):299–306.
31. Ahn J, Sinha R, Pei Z, et al. Human gut microbiome and risk for colorectal cancer. J Natl Cancer Inst 2013;105(24):1907–11.
32. Michaud DS. Role of bacterial infections in pancreatic cancer. Carcinogenesis 2013;34(10):2193–7.
33. Mitsuhashi K, Nosho K, Sukawa Y, et al. Association of *Fusobacterium* species in pancreatic cancer tissues with molecular features and prognosis. Oncotarget 2015;6(9):7209–20.
34. Fan X, Alekseyenko AV, Wu J, et al. Human oral microbiome and prospective risk for pancreatic cancer: a population-based nested case-control study. Gut 2018;67(1):120–7.
35. Karpiński TM. Role of oral microbiota in cancer development. Microorganisms 2019;7(1):20.
36. Raderer M, Wrba F, Kornek G, et al. Association between *Helicobacter pylori* infection and pancreatic cancer. Oncology 1998;55(1):16–9.
37. Stolzenberg-Solomon RZ, Blaser MJ, Limburg PJ, et al. *Helicobacter pylori* seropositivity as a risk factor for pancreatic cancer. J Natl Cancer Inst 2001;93:937–41.

38. Farrell JJ, Zhang L, Zhou H, et al. Variations of oral microbiota are associated with pancreatic diseases including pancreatic cancer. Gut 2012;61(4):582–8.

39. Lin IH, Wu J, Cohen SM, et al. Pilot study of oral microbiome and risk of pancreatic cancer [Abstract 101]. Cancer Res 2013;73(8):101.

40. Torres PJ, Fletcher EM, Gibbons SM, et al. Characterization of the salivary microbiome in patients with pancreatic cancer. PeerJ 2015;3:e1373.

41. Lu H, Ren Z, Li A, et al. Tongue coating microbiome data distinguish patients with pancreatic head cancer from healthy controls. J Oral Microbiol 2019; 11(1):1563409.

42. Del Castillo E, Meier R, Chung M, et al. The microbiomes of pancreatic and duodenum tissue overlap and are highly subject specific but differ between pancreatic cancer and noncancer subjects. Cancer Epidemiol Biomarkers Prev 2019;28(2):370–83.

43. Michaud DS, Izard J, Wilhelm-Benartzi CS, et al. Plasma antibodies to oral bacteria and risk of pancreatic cancer in a large European prospective cohort study. Gut 2013;62(12):1764–70.

44. Yamamura K, Baba Y, Miyake K, et al. *Fusobacterium nucleatum* in gastroenterological cancer: evaluation of measurement methods using quantitative polymerase chain reaction and a literature review. Oncol Lett 2017;14(6):6373–8.

45. Olson SH, Satagopan J, Xu Y, et al. The oral microbiota in patients with pancreatic cancer, patients with IPMNs, and controls: a pilot study. Cancer Causes Control 2017;28(9):959–69.

46. Half E, Keren N, Dorfman T, et al. Specific changes in fecal microbiota may differentiate pancreatic cancer patients from healthy individuals. Ann Oncol 2015;26:iv48.

47. Maekawa T, Fukaya R, Takamatsu S, et al. Possible involvement of *Enterococcus* infection in the pathogenesis of chronic pancreatitis and cancer. Biochem Biophys Res Commun 2018;506(4):962–9.

48. International Agency for Research on Cancer. Schistosomes, liver flukes and *Helicobacter pylori*. Evaluation of carcinogenic risks to humans. IARC Monogr Eval Carcinog Risks Hum 1994;61:177–240.

49. Karpiński TM, Andrzejewska E, Eder P, et al. Evaluation of antimicrobial resistance of *Helicobacter pylori* in the last 15 years in West Poland. Acta Microbiol Immunol Hung 2015;62(3):287–93.

50. Nilsson HO, Stenram U, Ihse I, et al. *Helicobacter* species ribosomal DNA in the pancreas, stomach and duodenum of pancreatic cancer patients. World J Gastroenterol 2006;12(19):3038–43.

51. Guo Y, Liu W, Wu J. *Helicobacter pylori* infection and pancreatic cancer risk: a meta-analysis. J Cancer Res Ther 2016;12(Supplement):C229e32.

52. Xiao M, Wang Y, Gao Y. Association between *Helicobacter pylori* infection and pancreatic cancer development: a meta-analysis. PLoS One 2013;8(9):e75559.

53. Trikudanathan G, Philip A, Dasanu CA, et al. Association between *Helicobacter pylori* infection and pancreatic cancer. A cumulative meta-analysis. JOP 2011; 12(1):26–31.

54. Gawin A, Wex T, Lawniczak M, et al. *Helicobacter pylori* infection in pancreatic cancer (in Polish). Pol Merkur Lekarski 2012;32:103–7.

55. Liu H, Chen YT, Wang R, et al. *Helicobacter pylori* infection, atrophic gastritis, and pancreatic cancer risk: a meta-analysis of prospective epidemiologic studies. Medicine (Baltimore) 2017;96(33):e7811.

56. Schulte A, Pandeya N, Fawcett J, et al. Association between *Helicobacter pylori* and pancreatic cancer risk: a meta-analysis. Cancer Causes Control 2015; 26(7):1027–35.

57. Wang Y, Zhang FC, Wang YJ. *Helicobacter pylori* and pancreatic cancer risk: a meta-analysis based on 2,049 cases and 2,861 controls. Asian Pac J Cancer Prev 2014;15(11):4449–54.

58. Chen XZ, Wang R, Chen HN, et al. Cytotoxin-associated gene a-negative strains of *Helicobacter pylori* as a potential risk factor of pancreatic cancer: a meta-analysis based on nested case-control studies. Pancreas 2015;44(8):1340–4.

59. Szkaradkiewicz AK, Karpiński TM. Microbiology of chronic periodontitis. J Biol Earth Sci 2013;3(1):M14–20.

60. Ochi A, Nguyen AH, Bedrosian AS, et al. MyD88 inhibition amplifies dendritic cell capacity to promote pancreatic carcinogenesis via Th2 cells. J Exp Med 2012;209:1671–87.

61. Hoque R, Mehal WZ. Inflammasomes in pancreatic physiology and disease. Am J Physiol Gastrointest Liver Physiol 2015;308(8):G643–51.

62. Hou LT, Liu CM, Liu BY, et al. Interleukin-1β, clinical parameters and matched cellular-histopathologic changes of biopsied gingival tissue from periodontitis patients. J Periodontal Res 2003;38:247–54.

63. Konopka Ł, Brzezińska-Błaszczyk E. Cytokines in gingival crevicular fluid as potential diagnostic and prognostic markers of periodontitis. Dent Med Probl 2010; 47(2):206–13.

64. Carmi Y, Dotan S, Rider P, et al. The role of IL-1β in the early tumor cell-induced angiogenic response. J Immunol 2013;190(7):3500–9.

65. Voronov E, Shouval DS, Krelin Y, et al. IL-1 is required for tumor invasiveness and angiogenesis. Proc Natl Acad Sci U S A 2003;100(5):2645–50.

66. Wang FM, Liu HQ, Liu SR, et al. SHP-2 promoting migration and metastasis of MCF-7 with loss of E-cadherin, dephosphorylation of FAK and secretion of MMP-9 induced by IL-1beta in vivo and in vitro. Breast Cancer Res Treat 2005;89:5–14.

67. Mathy-Hartert M, Hogge L, Sanchez C, et al. Interleukin-1beta and interleukin-6 disturb the antioxidant enzyme system in bovine chondrocytes: a possible explanation for oxidative stress generation. Osteoarthritis Cartilage 2008; 16(7):756–63.

68. Murata M, Thanan R, Ma N, et al. Role of nitrative and oxidative DNA damage in inflammation-related carcinogenesis. J Biomed Biotechnol 2012;2012:623019.

69. Haura EB, Turkson J, Jove R. Mechanisms of disease: insights into the emerging role of signal transducers and activators of transcription in cancer. Nat Clin Pract Oncol 2005;2(6):315–24.

70. Mei QX, Huang CL, Luo SZ, et al. Characterization of the duodenal bacterial microbiota in patients with pancreatic head cancer vs. healthy controls. Pancreatology 2018;18(4):438–45.

71. Bradley JR. TNF-mediated inflammatory disease. J Pathol 2008;214:149–60.

72. Szlosarek P, Charles KA, Balkwill FR. Tumour necrosis factor-alpha as a tumour promoter. Eur J Cancer 2006;42(6):745–50.

73. Rivas MA, Carnevale RP, Proietti CJ, et al. TNF alpha acting on TNFR1 promotes breast cancer growth via p42/P44 MAPK, JNK, Akt and NF-kappa B-dependent pathways. Exp Cell Res 2008;314(3):509–629.

74. Yoshida S, Ono M, Shono T, et al. Involvement of interleukin-8, vascular endothelial growth factor, and basic fibroblast growth factor in tumor necrosis factor alpha-dependent angiogenesis. Mol Cell Biol 1997;17(7):4015–23.

75. Leber TM, Balkwill FR. Regulation of monocyte MMP-9 production by TNF-alpha and a tumour-derived soluble factor (MMPSF). Br J Cancer 1998;78(6):724–32.
76. Landskron G, De la Fuente M, Thuwajit P, et al. Chronic inflammation and cytokines in the tumor microenvironment. J Immunol Res 2014;2014:149185.
77. Mittal M, Siddiqui MR, Tran K, et al. Reactive oxygen species in inflammation and tissue injury. Antioxid Redox Signal 2014;20(7):1126–67.
78. Abranches J, Zeng L, Kajfasz JK, et al. Biology of oral streptococci. Microbiol Spectr 2018;6(5). https://doi.org/10.1128/microbiolspec.GPP3-0042-2018.
79. Huycke MM, Moore D, Joyce W, et al. Extracellular superoxide production by *Enterococcus faecalis* requires demethylmenaquinone and is attenuated by functional terminal quinol oxidases. Mol Microbiol 2001;42:729–40.
80. Yilmaz Ö, Jungas T, Verbeke P, et al. Activation of the phosphatidylinositol 3-kinase/Akt pathway contributes to survival of primary epithelial cells infected with the periodontal pathogen *Porphyromonas gingivalis*. Infect Immun 2004;72(7): 3743–51.
81. Mao S, Park Y, Hasegawa Y, et al. Intrinsic apoptotic pathways of gingival epithelial cells modulated by Porphyromonas gingivalis. Cell Microbiol 2007; 9(8):1997–2007.
82. Whitmore SE, Lamont RJ. Oral bacteria and cancer. PLoS Pathog 2014;10(3): e1003933.
83. Yao L, Jermanus C, Barbetta B, et al. *Porphyromonas gingivalis* infection sequesters pro-apoptotic Bad through Akt in primary gingival epithelial cells. Mol Oral Microbiol 2010;25(2):89–101.
84. Nakhjiri SF, Park Y, Yilmaz O, et al. Inhibition of epithelial cell apoptosis by *Porphyromonas gingivalis*. FEMS Microbiol Lett 2001;200(2):145–9.
85. Inaba H, Sugita H, Kuboniwa M, et al. *Porphyromonas gingivalis* promotes invasion of oral squamous cell carcinoma through induction of proMMP9 and its activation. Cell Microbiol 2014;16(1):131–45.
86. Ögrendik M. Oral bacteria in pancreatic cancer: mutagenesis of the p53 tumour suppressor gene. Int J Clin Exp Pathol 2015;8:11835.
87. Liu L, Wang K, Zhu ZM, et al. Associations between P53 Arg72Pro and development of digestive tract cancers: a meta-analysis. Arch Med Res 2011; 42:60–9.
88. Spooner R, Yilmaz O. The role of reactive-oxygen-species in microbial persistence and inflammation. Int J Mol Sci 2011;12:334–52.
89. Baqui A, Meiller TF, Chon JJ, et al. Granulocyte-macrophage colony-stimulating factor amplification of interleukin-1b and tumor necrosis factor alpha production in THP-1 human monocytic cells stimulated with lipopolysaccharide of oral microorganisms. Clin Diagn Lab Immunol 1998;5(3):341–7.
90. Fischman S, Revach B, Bulvik R, et al. Periodontal pathogens *Porphyromonas gingivalis* and *Fusobacterium nucleatum* promote tumor progression in an oral-specific chemical carcinogenesis model. Oncotarget 2015;6(26):22613–23.
91. Rubinstein MR, Wang X, Liu W, et al. *Fusobacterium nucleatum* promotes colorectal carcinogenesis by modulating E-cadherin/b-catenin signaling via its FadA adhesin. Cell Host Microbe 2013;14(2):195–206.
92. Park HE, Kim JH, Cho NY, et al. Intratumoral *Fusobacterium nucleatum* abundance correlates with macrophage infiltration and CDKN2A methylation in microsatellite-unstable colorectal carcinoma. Virchows Arch 2017;471:329–36.
93. Chen Y, Peng Y, Yu J, et al. Invasive *Fusobacterium nucleatum* activates beta-catenin signaling in colorectal cancer via a TLR4/P-PAK1 cascade. Oncotarget 2017;8(19):31802–14.

94. Wu Y, Wu J, Chen T, et al. *Fusobacterium nucleatum* potentiates intestinal tumorigenesis in mice via a Toll-like receptor 4/p21-activated kinase 1 cascade. Dig Dis Sci 2018;63(5):1210–8.

95. Uitto VJ, Baillie D, Wu Q, et al. *Fusobacterium nucleatum* increases collagenase 3 production and migration of epithelial cells. Infect Immun 2005;73(2):1171–9.

96. Koczorowski R, Karpiński TM, Hofman J. Badanie zależności między halitosis a chorobami przyzębia. A study of the relationship between halitosis and periodontal diseases (in Polish). Dent Forum 2004;30(1):51–6.

97. Milella L. The negative effects of volatile sulphur compounds. J Vet Dent 2015; 32(2):99–102.

98. Attene-Ramos MS, Wagner ED, Plewa MJ, et al. Evidence that hydrogen sulfide is a genotoxic agent. Mol Cancer Res 2006;4(1):9–14.

99. Hellmich MR, Szabo C. Hydrogen sulfide and cancer. Handb Exp Pharmacol 2015;230:233–41.

100. Hooper SJ, Crean SJ, Fardy MJ, et al. A molecular analysis of the bacteria present within oral squamous cell carcinoma. J Med Microbiol 2007;56(Pt 12): 1651–9.

101. Karpiński TM, Szkaradkiewicz AK. Bacteriocins. In: Caballero B, Finglas PM, Toldra F, editors. Encyclopedia of food and health, vol. 1. Oxford (England): Elsevier; Academic Press; 2016. p. 312–9.

102. Lunt SJ, Chaudary N, Hill RP. The tumor microenvironment and metastatic disease. Clin Exp Metastasis 2009;26(1):19–34.

103. Mazzio E, Smith B, Soliman K. Evaluation of endogenous acidic metabolic products associated with carbohydrate metabolism in tumor cells. Cell Biol Toxicol 2010;26(3):177–88.

104. Pavlova SI, Jin L, Gasparovich SR, et al. Multiple alcohol dehydrogenases but no functional acetaldehyde dehydrogenase causing excessive acetaldehyde production from ethanol by oral streptococci. Microbiology 2013;159(Pt 7): 1437–46.

105. Marttila E, Bowyer P, Sanglard D, et al. Fermentative 2-carbon metabolism produces carcinogenic levels of acetaldehyde in *Candida albicans*. Mol Oral Microbiol 2013;28(4):281–91.

106. Muto M, Hitomi Y, Ohtsu A, et al. Acetaldehyde production by non-pathogenic *Neisseria* in human oral microflora: implications for carcinogenesis in upper aerodigestive tract. Int J Cancer 2000;88(3):342–50.

107. Wroblewski LE, Peek RM Jr. *Helicobacter pylori* in gastric carcinogenesis: mechanisms. Gastroenterol Clin North Am 2013;42:285–98.

108. Koeppel M, Garcia-Alcalde F, Glowinski F, et al. *Helicobacter pylori* infection causes characteristic DNA damage patterns in human cells. Cell Rep 2015; 11:1703–13.

109. O'Hara AM, Bhattacharyya A, Bai J. Tumor necrosis factor (TNF)-α-induced IL-8 expression in gastric epithelial cells: role of reactive oxygen species and AP endonuclease-1/redox factor (Ref)-1. Cytokine 2009;46:359–69.

110. Tsugawa H, Suzuki H, Saya H. Reactive oxygen species-induced autophagic degradation of *Helicobacter pylori* CagA is specifically suppressed in cancer stem-like cells. Cell Host Microbe 2012;12:764–77.

111. Butcher LD, den Hartog G, Ernst PB, et al. Oxidative stress resulting from *Helicobacter pylori* infection contributes to gastric carcinogenesis. Cell Mol Gastroenterol Hepatol 2017;3(3):316–22.

112. Kidane D. Molecular mechanisms of *H. pylori*-induced DNA double-strand breaks. Int J Mol Sci 2018;19(10) [pii:E2891].

113. Bartchewsky W Jr, Martini MR, Masiero M, et al. Effect of *Helicobacter pylori* infection on IL-8, IL-1beta and COX-2 expression in patients with chronic gastritis and gastric cancer. Scand J Gastroenterol 2009;44(2):153–61.

114. Kim JM, Kim JS, Lee JY. Vacuolating cytotoxin in *Helicobacter pylori* water-soluble proteins upregulates chemokine expression in human eosinophils via Ca^{2+} influx, mitochondrial reactive oxygen intermediates, and NF-κB activation. Infect Immun 2007;75:3373–81.

115. Risch HA. Etiology of pancreatic cancer, with a hypothesis concerning the role of N-nitroso compounds and excess gastric acidity. J Natl Cancer Inst 2003;95:948–96.

116. Kokkinakis DM, Reddy MK, Norgle JR, et al. Metabolism and activation of pancreas specific nitrosamines by pancreatic ductal cells in culture. Carcinogenesis 1993;14:1705–9.

117. Houben GM, Stockbrugger RW. Bacteria in the aetio-pathogenesis of gastric cancer: a review. Scand J Gastroenterol Suppl 1995;212:13–8.

118. Jin Y, Gao H, Chen H, et al. Identification and impact of hepatitis B virus DNA and antigens in pancreatic cancer tissues and adjacent non-cancerous tissues. Cancer Lett 2013;335(2):447–54.

119. Ben Q, Li Z, Liu C, et al. Hepatitis B virus status and risk of pancreatic ductal adenocarcinoma: a case-control study from China. Pancreas 2012;41:435–40.

120. Li L, Wu B, Yang LB, et al. Chronic hepatitis B virus infection and risk of pancreatic cancer: a meta-analysis. Asian Pac J Cancer Prev 2013;14(1):275–9.

121. Wang Y, Yang SI, Song FJ, et al. Hepatitis B virus status and the risk of pancreatic cancer: a meta-analysis. Eur J Cancer Prev 2013;22(4):328–34.

122. Luo G, Hao NB, Hu CJ, et al. HBV infection increases the risk of pancreatic cancer: a meta-analysis. Cancer Causes Control 2013;24(3):529–37.

123. Majumder S, Bockorny B, Baker WL, et al. Association between HBsAg positivity and pancreatic cancer: a meta-analysis. J Gastrointest Cancer 2014;45(3):347–52.

124. Xing S, Li ZW, Tian YF, et al. Chronic hepatitis virus infection increases the risk of pancreatic cancer: a meta-analysis. Hepatobiliary Pancreat Dis Int 2013;12:575–83.

125. Andersen ES, Omland LH, Jepsen P, et al. Risk of all-type cancer, hepatocellular carcinoma, non-Hodgkin lymphoma and pancreatic cancer in patients infected with hepatitis B virus. J Viral Hepat 2015;22(10):828–34.

126. Krull Abe S, Inoue M, Sawada N, et al. Hepatitis B and C virus infection and risk of pancreatic cancer: a population-based cohort study (JPHC Study Cohort II). Cancer Epidemiol Biomarkers Prev 2016;25(3):555–7.

127. Huang J, Magnusson M, Törner A, et al. Risk of pancreatic cancer among individuals with hepatitis C or hepatitis B virus infection: a nationwide study in Sweden. Br J Cancer 2013;109(11):2917–23.

128. Fiorino S, Chili E, Bacchi-Reggiani L, et al. Association between hepatitis B or hepatitis C virus infection and risk of pancreatic adenocarcinoma development: a systematic review and meta-analysis. Pancreatology 2013;2:147–60.

129. Takeda H, Takai A, Inuzuka T, et al. Genetic basis of hepatitis virus-associated hepatocellular carcinoma: linkage between infection, inflammation, and tumorigenesis. J Gastroenterol 2017;52(1):26–38.

130. Rajagopala SV, Vashee S, Oldfield LM, et al. The human microbiome and cancer. Cancer Prev Res (Phila) 2017;10(4):226–34.

131. Wang Z, Li Z, Ye Y, et al. Oxidative stress and liver cancer: etiology and therapeutic targets. Oxid Med Cell Longev 2016;2016:7891574.

132. Fiorino S, Cuppini A, Castellani G, et al. HBV- and HCV-related infections and risk of pancreatic cancer. JOP 2013;14(6):603–9.
133. Rossner MT. Review: hepatitis B virus X-gene product: a promiscuous transcriptional activator. J Med Virol 1992;36:101–17.
134. Su F, Schneider RJ. Hepatitis B virus HBx protein activates transcription factor NF-kappaB by acting on multiple cytoplasmic inhibitors of rel-related proteins. J Virol 1996;70:4558–66.
135. Yeh CT. Hepatitis B virus X protein: searching for a role in hepatocarcinogenesis. J Gastroenterol Hepatol 2000;15:339–41.
136. Waris G, Siddiqui A. Regulatory mechanisms of viral hepatitis B and C. J Biosci 2003;28:311–21.
137. Becker SA, Lee TH, Butel JS, et al. Hepatitis B virus X protein interferes with cellular DNA repair. J Virol 1998;72:266–72.
138. Takada S, Kaneniwa N, Tsuchida N, et al. Cytoplasmic retention of the p53 tumor suppressor gene product is observed in the hepatitis B virus X gene-transfected cells. Oncogene 1997;15:1895–901.
139. Ikeda K, Saitoh S, Koida I, et al. A multivariate analysis of risk factors for hepatocellular carcinogenesis: a prospective observation of 795 patients with viral and alcoholic cirrhosis. Hepatology 1993;18:47–53.
140. Lai MM, Ware CF. Hepatitis C virus core protein: possible roles in viral pathogenesis. Curr Top Microbiol Immunol 2000;242:117–34.
141. Okuda M, Li K, Beard MR, et al. Mitochondrial injury, oxidative stress, and antioxidant gene expression are induced by hepatitis C virus core protein. Gastroenterology 2002;122:366–75.
142. Kwun HJ, Jang KL. Dual effects of hepatitis C virus core protein on the transcription of cyclin-dependent kinase inhibitor p21 gene. J Viral Hepat 2003;10:249–55.
143. Kwun HJ, Jung EY, Ahn JY, et al. p53-dependent transcriptional repression of p21(waf1) by hepatitis C virus NS3. J Gen Virol 2001;82(Pt 9):2235–41.
144. Reyes GR. The nonstructural NS5A protein of hepatitis C virus: an expanding, multifunctional role in enhancing hepatitis C virus pathogenesis. J Biomed Sci 2002;9:187–97.
145. Zambirinis CP, Pushalkar S, Saxena D, et al. Pancreatic cancer, inflammation, and microbiome. Cancer J 2014;20(3):195–202.

Moving?

Make sure your subscription moves with you!

To notify us of your new address, find your **Clinics Account Number** (located on your mailing label above your name), and contact customer service at:

Email: journalscustomerservice-usa@elsevier.com

800-654-2452 (subscribers in the U.S. & Canada)
314-447-8871 (subscribers outside of the U.S. & Canada)

Fax number: 314-447-8029

Elsevier Health Sciences Division
Subscription Customer Service
3251 Riverport Lane
Maryland Heights, MO 63043

*To ensure uninterrupted delivery of your subscription, please notify us at least 4 weeks in advance of move.

Printed and bound by CPI Group (UK) Ltd, Croydon, CR0 4YY

03/10/2024

01040402-0015